The Business Side of Medicine:

A Survival Primer for Medical Students and Residents

By Ronald P. Kaufman, MD, FACPE

An ACPE Publication

American College of Physician Executives
Suite 200
4890 West Kennedy Boulevard
Tampa. Florida 33609
813/287-2000

ISBN: 0-924674-72-5
Library of Congress Card Number: 99-62644

Printed in the United States of America by Hillsboro Printing Company,
Tampa, Florida

About the Author

Ronald P. Kaufman, MD, FACPE, is Executive Director of the University of South Florida Physicians Group; Director, Division of Medical Practice Management; and Professor of Medicine at the University of South Florida College of Medicine, Tampa, Florida. He served as Vice President for Health Sciences at the University of South Florida Health Sciences Center from 1987 to 1994. Dr. Kaufman formerly held the positions of Vice President for Medical Affairs, Executive Dean, Walter A. Bloedorn Professor of Administrative Medicine, and Professor of Medicine at the George Washington University School of Medicine and Health Sciences, Washington, D.C., and Medical Director of the University Hospital, Associate Dean, Dean for Clinical Affairs, and Acting Vice President for Medical Affairs at the George Washington University Medical Center, Washington, D.C.

Dr. Kaufman earned his medical degree from the University of Pennsylvania School of Medicine and completed his internship and residency in internal medicine at Hartford (Connecticut) Hospital, where he served as Director of the Department of Medical Education.

He serves on a number of national committees and professional organizations and societies. He is a past member and Chairman of the Board of Directors of the Association of Academic Health Centers. He is a Fellow of the American College of Physician Executives (ACPE), and has served as President of both ACPE and the American Board of Medical Management.

Acknowledgments

In 1994, the University of South Florida College of Medicine recognized the need to inform its trainees, that is, medical students as well as residents, about major changes that were occurring in the organization and financing of health care and about how these changes would effect how medicine is practiced. Over time, a series of both didactic and interactive curricular offerings were developed and integrated within the basic medical school curriculum and as part of resident training programs. These offerings evolved into the material that created the basis for this book. Roger Schenke, Executive Vice President of the American College of Physicians Executives, encouraged me to put this material together as a basic primer, thereby creating a textbook for potential utilization in medical education throughout the United States. This volume essentially represents the culmination of that effort.

A number of individuals were critical in turning this concept into reality. They are Dr. Michael Alberts, who created the chapter on Quality; Mr. Bryan Burgess, who developed a very difficult chapter relative to the legal environment of medicine; Donna Vavala, who collated and integrated the information into a text; Ms. Betsy Willard, who was patient with the recurring requirements of frequent editing of the transcripts; and Elaine Phelps, who worked diligently on the illustrations.

Also, I want to sincerely thank my wife Beth for her patience and encouragement during this somewhat long and occasionally exasperating process.

Ronald P. Kaufman, MD, FACPE
University of South Florida
Tampa, Florida
June 1999

Table of Contents

Prologue

Introduction and Historical Evolution of Health Care in the United States

For better or worse, you are preparing to be physicians and to enter the medical profession in a very interesting, if somewhat unsettling, time. The medical profession is currently going through significant turbulence and instability. These major changes in health care are a consequence of a significant change in the organization and financing of health care, which affects how medicine itself is practiced.

For the past 50 or 60 years, medical educators have focused most of their energy offering medical students a firm grounding in basic and clinical sciences so that those with MD or DO degrees would have the scientific competence to diagnose, treat, and otherwise care for patients. Following the receipt of degrees, almost all entered into graduated, progressive, clinical experiences with decreasing supervision and increasing independence in selected specialties, experiences that we call residency programs. Rarely, if ever, did we spend much energy or time exposing students or residents to how the medical profession was organized or financed. Rather, new physicians, upon completion of their residencies, entered into private practice—set up an office alone or with another group of physicians and learned the relatively simple economics of fee-for-service practice as they went along. Many of us in medical education no longer believe that such a relaxed approach is acceptable in view of the changing health care marketplace, which, without question, significantly affects the doctor/patient relationship. We sincerely believe we have a major responsibility to medical students and residents to help them comprehend and understand what is happening in health care, because it will indeed affect the rest of their lives—clerkship years; residency training; and, most profoundly, their future, professional practice.*

I think it is fair to say that most of us are very comfortable with the status quo and frequently do not wish to embrace change and all of the uncertainty that comes with it. I don't think that many people in the medical profession would say that they are enamored with managed care. They would more likely wish to maintain the current situation or, if that can't be

done, hope that the changes we are undergoing are merely a fad and that the pendulum will rapidly swing back to an earlier time. Nonetheless, an appreciation and perspective on the changing environment of health care payment is very critical, because physicians

---

*Simon, S., and others. "Views of Managed Care—A Survey of Students, Residents, Faculty, and Deans of Medical Schools in the United States." New England Journal of Medicine 340(12):928-36, March 25, 1999.

today, in my view, are relatively disadvantaged. They have lived in an unrealistic world, from a business perspective—that of fee-for-service practice and cost reimbursement—for enough years to strongly believe not only that it should be that way, but also that it is the best and only way. No other business that I know of has had the benefit of such a forgiving environment. Like it or not, and most of us don't, medicine is now moving into the real world of commerce. A real world that would be defined by business people with a simple phrase, "The market is always right." Most of us would take great umbrage at this definition, but I'm sure that what most of these business people mean is "the market is always right because there is nothing else!" In other words, the environment we face is the only environment that we have, and, therefore, our first task is to understand it and to deal with it in a realistic manner.

We physicians have a major responsibility to stop focusing our energies on fighting managed care and the other changes in the health care system. Instead, we must focus our energies and expend our efforts to ensure that the unique relationship between physician and patient is maintained, that the physician continues to be a patient advocate, and that quality is as much a part of the competitive health equation as cost.

In order to achieve these goals, it is necessary to educate us and to convince our colleagues that changes can be viewed as opportunities for the future and worked toward with optimism, rather than negativism and dread.

Most of us in academic medicine believe that, before one embraces a methodology to strategically plan and make behavioral change, it is best to fully understand and analyze the situation in order to react in an intelligent and studied manner, rather than in a purely intuitive approach. The basis of this assumption relative to change is the fact that physicians are trained in the scientific method; before they make decisions, they must have accurate data so that their decisions will be evidence-based. Successful physicians incorporate that process into their decision making and culture. The same approach must be applied to the issues that will be discussed in this book. We believe that, once the data and evidence are presented, a logic will evolve that will enable physicians at all levels to understand the necessity for change and to begin the acculturation necessary for effective practice in the emerging business environment. In this way, they can be effective as physicians and healers as well as succeed economically.

Ronald P. Kaufman, MD, FACPE
University of South Florida
Tampa, Florida
June 1999

CHAPTER 1

Changes Driving the Way Health Care Is Delivered

Without question, health care delivery and its financing are undergoing very rapid and massive transformation. These changes will affect all physicians, not only economically but, perhaps more important, in how they practice medicine. In view of these profound changes, it is critical to try to understand the issues and to work to maintain a high quality of professionalism in the new and emerging world. We need to stop ranting and raving; engaging in unfocused anger, frustration, and unhappiness; and yearning longingly for the "good old days."

There is a growing consensus that changes in the delivery of health care will continue unremittingly as a consequence of:

- Political pressure leading to legislative health care reform, as well as some incremental changes at the federal level.

- Fiscal pressure to balance the federal budget, which is why the Balanced Budget Act of 1997 was enacted. It will temporarily slow the rising costs of both Medicare and Medicaid, therefore delaying the predicted bankruptcy of Medicare Part A from approximately the year 2001 to around the year 2010, but the issue will then re-emerge.

It has been a given that, since World War II, the United States has had the best medical research and the best physicians and scientists in the world. As a consequence, most people feel this country also offers the best medical care in the world—so good, in fact, that, for many years, people from all around the world have come here for their care. In addition, many foreign physicians come to the United States for their education, especially in subspecialty training. If this is all true, what factors are pushing us inexorably toward significant modification in the way health care is delivered and financed?

Two major factors are the rapidly rising costs of health care and access to care. Bear in mind that these factors are, in reality, constantly intertwined. Since 1960, health care costs in the United States have been rising on a very steep curve and now consume approximately 13.5 percent of the Gross Domestic Product (GDP). In reaction to those rising costs, both private and public payers have taken steps to limit access and utilization.

THE BUSINESS SIDE OF MEDICINE:

A Survival Primer for Medical Students and Residents

Health Care Expenditures

Although absolute health care spending in the United States did increase, in 1996 topping the $1 trillion mark, cost control policies, especially through managed care and the low inflation rate, have slowed the rate of spending increases from close to 9 percent per year to less than 5 percent per year (figure 1, below). The 4.4 percent increase in 1996 was the slowest growth in health care since 1960. Health care costs, as a percentage of the GDP, are hovering around 13 percent (figure 2, page 3). Health care spending has been relatively flat, but still in excess of the Consumer Price Index (CPI).

Although national health care spending increases have been muted, spending is expected to reach nearly $1.5 trillion by the year 2002, unless some additional changes in the organization and the financing of health care occur. Physicians and hospitals directly consume approximately 60 percent of total expenditures in health care and, therefore, not surprisingly, are viewed as the areas in which health care spending must be constrained (figure 3, page 3).

In the past 25 years, personal health care spending more than doubled, from about 7 percent to some 18 percent, far exceeding what most Americans consider an appropriate

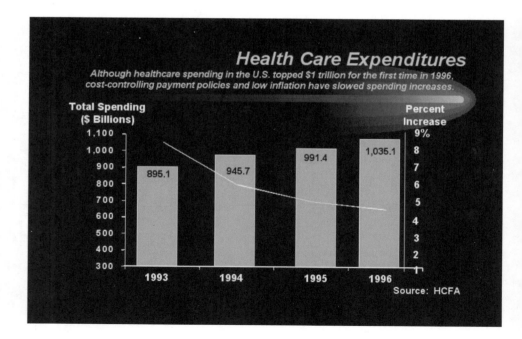

Figure 1

National Health Expenditure (NHE) Forecasts, 1996 to 2000

Year	1997 Estimates (dollars in billions)	Growth Rate	NHE as a percentage of GDP[1]
1996	$1,035.1	4.4%	13.6%
1997	1,096.4	5.9	13.6
1998	1,153.1	5.2	13.5
1999	1,221.3	5.9	13.5
2000	1,289.3	5.6	13.5

[1] Assumes real gross domestic product growth of 3% in 1998, 1999 and 2000. GDP is the total value of goods and services produced in the United States.

NOTE: These results are not stated on a per capita basis.

SOURCE: Cookson and Reilly, Milliman & Robertson, March, 1998

Figure 2

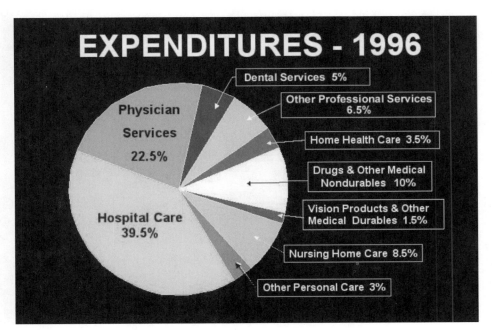

Figure 3

percentage of their discretionary spending. The United States significantly exceeds all industrialized nations in the percentage of GDP expended on health care (figure 4, below). Health care here is by far the most expensive in the world. And the gap between this country and other industrialized nations is widening. The bottom line is that the majority of other industrialized nations have managed to slow the growth of health care costs over the past 10 years, whereas the U.S. has not. In fact, in 1997, average per capita spending in the United States was $4,090 per person, or more than a $1,000 increase since 1991 (figure 5, page 5)

Another broad issue is the impact that health care costs have on the general economy. Major employers, especially those, such as the automotive industry, that compete internationally, have become increasingly concerned about health care costs and what they add to the cost of their products and how they affect their ability to compete internationally.

There has been a growing gap between U.S. medical costs and global sales prices. This large gap, which is predicted to significantly increase in the next few years, represents the costs that are imbedded in the prices of U.S. products sold abroad. This is a cause of significant concern to the U.S. economy, which, as we all know, is international and not merely local.

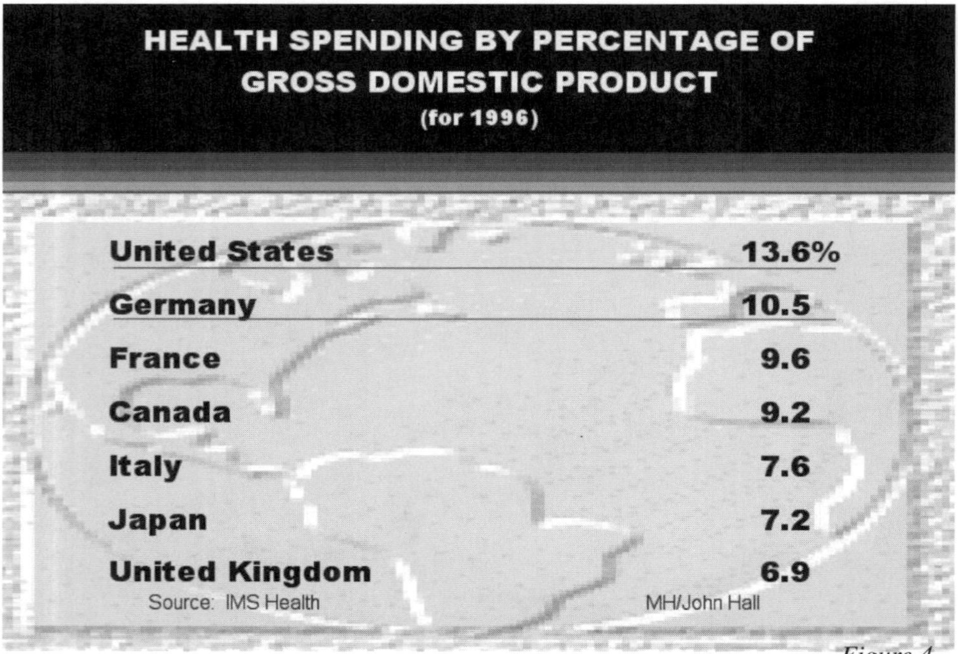

HEALTH SPENDING BY PERCENTAGE OF GROSS DOMESTIC PRODUCT
(for 1996)

United States	13.6%
Germany	10.5
France	9.6
Canada	9.2
Italy	7.6
Japan	7.2
United Kingdom	6.9

Source: IMS Health   MH/John Hall

Figure 4

Major Forces Fueling Inflationary Spiral

The major forces fueling health care cost inflation include:

- U.S. demographic changes, especially the aging of America—the rapidly growing portion of the population over 65 years of age.

- Major societal problems, such as drug use, cigarette smoking, alcohol abuse, and crime and trauma related to the broad use of handguns and automatic weapons.

- Charges and demonstration of waste/fraud and abuse within the health care administrative structure, accounting, by some estimates, for up to 15 percent of total costs.

- Physician behavior, including:

  - Defensive medicine—fear and subsequent actions taken by physicians because of concern about malpractice, which is estimated to cost about $50 billion per year.

  - Increased use of high technology. In theory, some technological

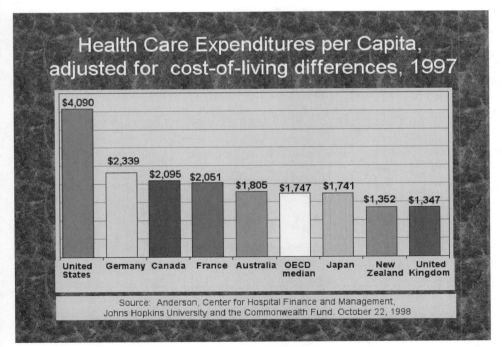

Figure 5

advantages should be translated into cost savings. However, in the long term, most technological advances translate into higher costs. It is not difficult for us to imagine the significant incremental costs that will accompany implementation of genetic therapies when applied to the bedside, whether it is in cystic fibrosis, diabetes, obesity, Alzheimer's disease, or other diseases and conditions.

○ The more is better syndrome. Medical educators have spent the past 50 years ingraining into physicians that more information is better—that doing more is better. The basic concept is that, when you hear hoof beats, it cannot possibly be horses; one must always look for zebras.

○ The degree of diagnostic uncertainty or confidence with which any individual physician can live. Is the performance of another diagnostic test or procedure, although it increases the physician's confidence by a small percentage, worth the incremental cost?

How Physicians Have Been Historically Paid

Prior to 1910, there was no truly scientifically based care for individuals. Most of the really effective health care that was available was in the public health sector. Disease was controlled primarily by means of public sanitation relative to food handling, the water supply, and insect and vermin control. In this manner, public health successes occurred in curbing illness such as malaria, tuberculosis, and the plague. In this era, any encounter with a physician was a very dangerous event for a patient. There was no better than a 50/50 chance of being helpful, because the armamentaria of physicians were limited to utilization of opiates, bleeding, leeching, and the like.

In 1910, Abraham Flexner produced his now famous report on medical education, which, without exaggeration, revolutionized medicine. Marginal proprietary medical schools were closed. In parallel, there began to be created a scientific basis for the practice of medicine out of which flowed creation of the basic medical school curriculum, the core of which is still followed today in broad strokes. Almost all medical school curricula begin with the basic sciences so that practicing physicians can apply understanding of the human body and its pathology to clinical situations that present themselves.

In the first half of the 20th Century, physicians were not well compensated and were often not well respected. They were not infrequently referred to as "quacks" and were only utilized as a last resort in many cases. Hospitals were feared, because they were not institutions one went to get well, but rather places where people were sent to die or, at best, to be confined for tuberculosis or for mental disorders. There still is reason for concern today, because approximately 18 percent of hospitalizations include a very serious adverse event.

During the decade of 1940-1950, two major societal interventions occurred, almost in parallel and, perhaps, causally related. First, there was a significant increase in understanding of the scientific method related to medical research. As a consequence, there was an increase in scientific information that had direct applicability to individual patients. This resulted in the discovery of antimicrobials, such as the sulfonimides and penicillin. There was also a great increase in the use of aseptic techniques in general surgery. Last, there was the emergence of research funded by the federal government through the National Institutes of Health and by private industry in both the United States and abroad.

The second societal intervention was major and significant change in payment methodologies for individual health care. An appreciation of the historic perspective relative to these payment methodologies can help one understand why we are where we are and where we are going. This historical view can also help in acceptance of the rationale behind current and future changes in payment methodologies.

Methods of Payment for Personal Health Care

From a medical economics perspective, there are essentially four primary modes of payment for personal health care services

- Out of Pocket.
- Individual Private Insurance.
- Employment-Based Private Group Insurance.
- Government-Financed Coverage.

Out of Pocket—19 Percent

As mentioned earlier, during the first half of the 20th Century, physicians were not well compensated. In less urban areas, they often got paid by the barter method—having their roofs fixed; having their vehicles repaired; or being plied with chickens, eggs, etc. in return for a specific service. In addition to barter, of course, there was payment by cash, out-of-pocket, as some sort of fee that was set in a very loose and uncontrolled manner.

What is wrong with this? This is the way we pay for most commodities. If we intend to buy a car, a television set, a portable phone, a personal computer, a VCR, etc., we decide what we can afford, we shop for a good price, and then we decide whether we're going to purchase it or not. This works fine in most of the economy, because, other than commodities such as food and shelter, consumer items are relatively optional. This is not always true with health care. It is not always optional and, indeed, is often considered by some to be a basic human need. Also, unlike for other commodities, the need for health care is often unpredictable and the cost itself, if catastrophic, can be devastating to the individual. Although highly unattractive, out-of-pocket payment is still a methodology for payment of health care, especially for the rich and for the unemployed and poor.

Individual Private Insurance—4 Percent

Individual private insurance is analogous to automobile insurance, life insurance, or homeowner insurance. Although such an approach makes sense and is used in some parts of industrialized Europe, such as Germany, it has not become a popular method of payment in the United States because of the high costs and the administrative burden of collecting and monitoring individual premiums. However, the 104th Congress began rethinking this approach, using the terms "vouchers" or "medical savings accounts," in proposing expansion of individual private insurance in enactment of the Health Insurance Portability and Accountability Act of 1996, the Kassebaum-Kennedy Bill.

Employment-Based Insurance—31 Percent

Employment-based private insurance has been, and continues to be, the most prominent methodology, other than government programs, for payment for personal health care in the United States. Employment-based insurance and its preservation seem to be the cornerstone of all political debates and discussions in the United States. In the late 1930s and 1940s, when hospitals suddenly became places for successful treatments and not merely custodial places for individuals to be warehoused or to die, they were expensive. Hospitals thought it would be in their best interests to get into the insurance business and to make their product more attractive, affordable, and readily accessible. So the American Hospital Association, in the late 1930s and early 1940s, began an insurance program that it called Blue Cross to reimburse hospitals for their expenses. Physicians saw the attractiveness of such an approach, and not wanting to be left out of the mix, began a program they called Blue Shield, a prepayment insurance program to cover physicians' services.

Through the Blue Cross/Blue Shield approach, a major societal divergence from the health care methodology being followed in other industrialized nations occurred. In other industrialized nations, consumer-driven, societal health reform focused on creating a socialized good. In the United States, on the other hand, insurance has been provider-driven in order to create a steady stream of income to allow patients to have access to doctors and hospitals utilizing Blue Cross/Blue Shield. Not surprisingly, because Blue Cross and Blue Shield were initially hospital- and doctor-controlled, reimbursement was very generous, and cost controls were not part of the equation.

The lack of cost sensitivity in employment-based insurance was compounded during

World War II because of a major historical fluke. As part of the war effort, the United States imposed effective wage and price controls on all industries. However, there was no related restriction on fringe benefits. Therefore, fringe benefits, especially health benefits through employment, grew. After World War II, labor unions picked up on this concept and made it part of their bargaining with employers. In parallel, and significantly, the federal government decided that employer premiums were to be tax deductible business expenditures to the employer and decided to treat health insurance fringe benefits as a tax deductible item to the individual employee. Herein lies the firm cornerstone of today's health care financing in the United States: employment-based and exempt from taxes for employer and employee.

With the explosion of employment-based health insurance, a significant and major modification of the financial transaction in health care developed. As noted before, a simple transaction in most commodities is between two parties. In health care, those two parties are the patient and the physician, or the patient and the hospital. In the insurance model, especially in the employment-based insurance model, there is a third party. Thus, the derivation of the term "third-party payer" or "third-party insurer."

So, with the introduction and explosion of insurance, there was a new dynamic. First was the third-party nature of the transaction. Another element was the basic concept of any health insurance: nonusers of insurance pay for the users. In health insurance, of course, the healthy pay for the sick. Spread over an entire population, this is called "community rating," which is conducted without any regard to risk or pre-existing conditions. On the other end of the scale is what is called "experience rating." This is far less redistributive, because low-risk individuals don't subsidize high-risk individuals. In the United States, we have gradually moved from "community rating" under early Blue Cross/Blue Shield plans more to "experience rating" once the market heats up. There is now, however, a push under health care reform to return to "community rating" or "modified community rating" in order to again redistribute health care costs in a "more equitable manner."

Health insurance, especially employer-based health insurance, had thus become the major social intervention to achieve more universal access to health care and to cover its basic costs. However, in solving that problem, we created new problems. Utilizing the passive third-party insurance approach stimulated a rapid rise in health care costs. The user (patient) is highly insulated from the price/cost of the commodity (health care). Moreover, in a hospital- and physician-controlled insurer system such as Blue Cross/Blue Shield, reimbursement to hospitals and physicians also rose. And, as we moved from "community rating" to "experience rating," low-income individuals, the chronically ill, and the elderly began to fall between the cracks and became increasingly uninsurable. These situations stimulated the demand for federal intervention.

Government—46 Percent

With the growth of employment-based insurance, working Americans and dependents became more and more secure, but, as just mentioned, the poor and the elderly became more exposed and more at risk. The elderly became increasingly exposed with a decrease in community rating so that, in the 1950s, only 15 percent of individuals over 65 were covered by insurance. That stimulated great concern at the federal level and resulted, in 1965 under President Lyndon Johnson, in the passage of tax-based, government-financed health insurance programs called Medicare and Medicaid.

Medicare, the health care federal program for the elderly, has two parts. Part A, hospital insurance that is funded from Social Security taxes on both employers and employees, is the primary element of Medicare and was being projected to go into bankruptcy by the year 2001. As a consequence of these projections, the Congress and the Administration have significantly curtailed the growth of Medicare Part A as part of the legislation contained in the Balanced Budget Act of 1997.

Medicare Part B is payment for physician services and is funded from general taxes plus premiums collected from beneficiaries.

In addition, under the Balanced Budget Act of 1997, a new program, Medicare Plus Choice (Medicare Part C) was enacted.

Medicaid is a state-operated health care program for the poor and the disabled and is supported by federal and state taxes. Although Congress is considering major modifications to the Medicaid program, the action in Medicaid is primarily at the state level, where more and more states have requested and obtained waivers in order to shift Medicaid-eligible patients into managed care plans.

Through these rudimentary ABCs of how physicians and hospitals are paid, we have moved from out-of-pocket individual payments through an evolution of employment-based insurance and the entry of government into payment for health care. The combination of employment-based insurance and government payment makes up almost 80 percent of health care financing and has created some very new and very unexpected consequences.

The major consequence of employment-based insurance, tax-exempt treatment of health insurance, and the third-party nature of insurance itself, which insulates patients from fully experiencing the cost of health care as an element of the insurance transaction, has been an almost insatiable demand for health care. Concomitantly, runaway price increases that have driven up the cost of health care have been stimulated.

Access to Health Care

Based on the most recent U.S. Census Bureau estimates, the U.S. population is more than 270 million. Approximately 60 percent of the U.S. population is privately insured; approximately 25 percent is under some federal program, such as Medicare, Medicaid, or Champus (the military personnel and dependents program); and some 18 percent is uninsured. Since 1995, the number of uninsured has increased by approximately 4 million to some 43 million Americans, a rate of increase of approximately 1 million per year. Importantly, of the 43 million, more than 10 million are children (figure 6, below).

As a consequence, and closely interrelated with health care cost escalation, the problem of access has become more and more acute. As costs for health care have gone up, employers have progressively decreased health care benefits and added to the number of uninsured (figure 7, page 12). In the late 1980s, 61 percent of the population was insured by employers and 13 percent was uninsured. Today, nearly 25 percent of the American work force is employed by companies that do not offer group health insurance to their families. As employers drop their coverage, the number of uninsured has risen dramatically.

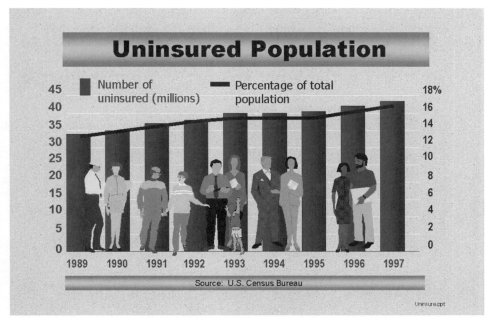

Figure 6

THE BUSINESS SIDE OF MEDICINE:
A Survival Primer for Medical Students and Residents

Identifying the Uninsured

The vast majority of uninsured are workers and their dependents, especially children, with nonworkers making up only about 18 percent of the distribution. A common misconception is that people without insurance are unemployed. As a consequence, the new political focus on access will be on the approximately 10 million children who do not have health insurance. In 1997, Congress began to address the issue of children without access to health care and has created some flexibility for the states to begin to develop their own programs relative to care of children. Most states have already begun planning such an initiative in the hope of significantly reducing this element of the uninsured population. Without question, the evidence is clear that children from families who do not have health insurance are far less likely to get medical care when they need it.

The Issue of Quality

Conventional wisdom has always assumed that the United States has the best quality of health care in the world, but, in many areas, this is not the case. A 1996 research study conducted by Market Line International[1] compared factors, such as per capita health care expenditures, number of doctors per capita, infant mortality rates, life expectancy, key

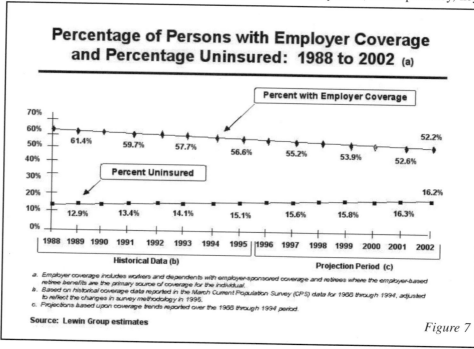

Percentage of Persons with Employer Coverage and Percentage Uninsured: 1988 to 2002 (a)

Percent with Employer Coverage

Percent Uninsured

61.4% 59.7% 57.7% 56.6% 55.2% 53.9% 52.6% 52.2%

12.9% 13.4% 14.1% 15.1% 15.6% 15.8% 16.3% 16.2%

1988 1989 1990 1991 1992 1993 1994 1995 | 1996 1997 1998 1999 2000 2001 2002

Historical Data (b)   Projection Period (c)

a. Employer coverage includes workers and dependents with employer-sponsored coverage and retirees where the employer-based retiree benefits are the primary source of coverage for the individual.
b. Based on historical coverage data reported in the March Current Population Survey (CPS) data for 1988 through 1994, adjusted to reflect the changes in survey methodology in 1995.
c. Projections based upon coverage trends reported over the 1988 through 1994 period.

Source: Lewin Group estimates

Figure 7

causes of death, and level of accessibility of health care services. Utilizing those criteria, countries were ranked relative to overall quality of health care. Switzerland was first, followed by Sweden, Austria, and Japan. The United States ranked number 12; Canada was 6; and the United Kingdom was 8. Looking at life expectancy, when last correlated in 1995, the United States reached a record high of 75.8 years (on average of male and female), compared with other industrialized nations, which are much closer to 79+ years. In addition, infant mortality in the U.S. hit a record low of 7.5 infant deaths-per-100,000 births. This, too, significantly exceeded the statistic for other industrialized nations, which ranged between 4.5 and 6.5 per 100,000. The researchers' conclusion was that the U.S. health system provides poor value for the money expended, while still leaving a significant number of the population without access to care.

Perception of Greed

Whether physician fees are justified or not, there is a general feeling that physicians are overpaid. In addition, there are data demonstrating a growing number of referrals of patients to diagnostic and treatment facilities owned by referring physicians. Whether this is appropriate or not is becoming immaterial, because it presents a perception of self-dealing on the part of physicians and has resulted in specific legislative action at the federal level, called Stark I and Stark II, to prohibit such activities. Significant changes in the Stark I and Stark II constraints were incorporated in the Health Insurance Portability and Accountability Act of 1996.

The Stark I and II regulations banning certain types of physician referrals were published in January 1998. Essentially, the rules prohibit physicians from making referrals to a number of entities in which they or their families have a financial stake— clinical laboratories; inpatient and outpatient hospital services; outpatient prescription drugs; home health services; durable medical equipment and supplies; radiation therapy services; and radiological services, including MRIs, CAT scans, and ultrasound services. The purpose of the law and the regulations is to prevent physicians from profiting from referral decisions. The violators face civil penalties of up to $15,000 per self-referred service.

In addition, there have been allegations of serious fraudulent activities, especially in the Medicare area, that have resulted in grand jury investigations of physician and hospital charges in a number of states.

The bottom line is that most polls confirm what we intuitively believe—that the vast majority of physicians are ethical and hardworking individuals who are well thought of by their personal patients and are primarily motivated to treat the ill. As a group, however, physicians have had their image significantly tarnished and are not held in the same high esteem they were in the recent past.

Five National Health Systems at a Glance

Why does the United States spend more money on health care and still have more disenfranchised individuals than other industrialized countries? This simple question has led to many in-depth studies of the health care systems of other industrialized nations and the United States, especially focusing on comparisons with Canada, Germany, Japan, the Netherlands, and the United Kingdom. All of these countries have broad-based individual coverage. The coverage often comes, as it does in the United States, from an employment base; most physician payments are based on a fee-for-service concept. The hospital sector, however, is usually controlled by a global budgeting process. And, of most significance, there is a major role played by government in all these programs. As a consequence of this latter element, such international approaches are labeled "socialized medicine."

This subject was very well addressed, in my view, by Odin Anderson[2] in a 1988 article. He conceptualizes placing the various nations on a market-minimized/market-maximized continuum. Anderson notes that, on that continuum, one would place the United Kingdom at the extreme of market-minimized, because the National Health Service in the United Kingdom is completely government-financed and operated. He placed the United States at the opposite extreme, the market-maximized pole of the continuum. According to Anderson, this country has been "cut loose in an open field in a way no other country has conceived of or dared to try." What he means is that other industrialized nations have chosen to look at health care as a service that must be available to the vast majority of its citizens and whose financing must, directly or indirectly, be through government. The United States chose a very different approach and decided that health protection was to come through employment-based insurance, the primary purpose of which was to protect providers so that they have the ability to bill and collect for their services.

Anderson suggests grouping international health care systems into three basic models:

- The National Health Services model is characterized by universal coverage, general national tax financing, and national ownership and/or control of the factors of production.

- The social insurance model, which is used by Germany and Japan, has compulsory universal coverage within a framework of social security and is financed by employer and individual contributions through not-for-profit insurance funds and public and/or private ownership of the factors of production.

- The U.S. private insurance model is characterized by employer-based or individual-purchased insurance, financed by individual and/or employer contributions, and private ownership of the factors of production.

It is very important to note that the continuum is not static and that there is constant narrowing of the gaps between the systems. Nonetheless, it is probable that any attempt to move to the left would be culturally resisted in the United States, because our democratic system is deeply routed in its decentralized nature. The health care systems found in other industrialized nations are deeply rooted in their trust of a centralized government organization with related funding mechanisms. A recent survey[3] revealed that:

- Americans are dissatisfied with their health care system but are still not disposed to involve the government.

- Canadians and Germans are experiencing increasing dissatisfaction with their health care systems but don't necessarily want to abandon their current health care systems.

General Domestic Strategies Available

With this as a backdrop, let us explore in a broad sense what options the United States might embrace as it moves forward to address the health care issues that still exist.

The Canadian health care system is a single-payer system. Some states have toyed with this idea, especially Vermont and, in a recently defeated referendum, California. Although there are some very strong advocates of a single payer approach, there is general belief that the U.S. public, with its long history of not trusting central government to do anything important, is in no way ready to embrace a single-payer, tax-based system at this time. Nonetheless, many people believe that this country will ultimately move toward such a system after attempting to make one or more of the market-based approaches work.

The vast majority of Canadians are still very pleased and comfortable with their health system, and very few would wish to switch to the U.S. approach, according to a relatively recent Gallop poll.[4] The Canadian system provides universal access, is not tied to employment, and is truly portable. There is free choice of physicians and hospitals, and physicians are paid on a fee-for-service basis.

The Canadian system has, in general, controlled overall costs and their rate of increase. Canada is now spending $73 billion per year on health care, which is only 9 percent of the Gross Domestic Product. Canada is no longer second to this country in the cost of delivering health care and now ranks seventh in the world, according to Hugh Scott, MD, Executive Director of the Royal College of Physicians and Surgeons, in Canada.[5] In addition, physicians in Canada and the United States are comparably compensated.

The downside is the well-publicized problem of queuing. However, some very good studies indicate that the queuing issue has been exaggerated to make a political point. Objective measurements of medical and surgical outcomes that compare the United States and Canada do not demonstrate any real variances in quality or outcome. Although the Canadian system is undergoing stress and the government is looking at increased financial control, its citizens are still overwhelmingly in favor of the country's single-payer national health care system (figure 8, below)

.

Median Waiting Times and Charges for Selected Procedures

Procedures	Waiting times (days) U.S.	Canada	Charges in U.S. currency U.S.	Canada
MRI of head	3	150	$ 1,218	$ 888
Mammogram	7	16	130	77
Electrocardiogram	1	1	97	23
Prothrombin time	1	1	25	8
Hemodialysis session	7	21	326	402
Screening colonoscopy	14	21	1,736	606
Total knee replacement	25	165	$26,805	$10,651

Source: Journal of the American Medical Association, 1998

Figure 8

Canada has been able to hold its costs relatively stable at approximately 10 percent of the gross domestic product. Moreover, the U.S. Congressional Budget Office estimates that, if the Canadian system were implemented in the United States today, it would save approximately $250 billion dollars as a consequence of reduction of administrative paperwork and other bureaucratic encumbrances.

Pay or Play

A popular health insurance option in the United States is usually referred to as "play or pay." The extension of our current employment-based health insurance methodology in the play or pay system is an employer mandate with an additional rule: An employer who does not cover workers must contribute to a government fund used to cover the uninsured. Oregon, for example, follows this approach to mandate employer provision of coverage. And the states of Washington and Massachusetts placed this feature in their health reform legislative packages.

There are a vast number of variations of the theme, but just two major approaches to look at:

- All employers must offer all employees a basic package of benefits or, as noted earlier, must buy an equivalent package from a government program. This is the pure form of "play or pay." It has lacked support, because it is predicted by many that small employers would opt for the pay option, and we would therefore, de facto, end up in the single-payer, Canadian-like system.

- The second and most popular approach, which has a number of further themes and variations, is encompassed under the managed competition rubric. This approach may or may not have linked with it expenditure limits, targets, or overall budgets. Essentially, this was the core of President Clinton's health reform proposal, which was soundly rejected.

Vouchers or Tax Credits

This is a concept of offering individuals vouchers or tax credits that they use to purchase health insurance. This approach has been promulgated by the Heritage Foundation and has been a favorite of conservatives, especially conservative Republicans. It has now re-emerged in Congress under the rubric of vouchers and medical savings accounts (MSAs).

The Open Market

The open-market concept is essentially a return to the early history of payment for health care. Although the open market does not have a set of advocates, many would state that the current market forces we are experiencing, with minimal government oversight, are becoming, de facto, the open-market concept or, as some refer to it, "The Industrialization of Medicine."

The current desire to constrain the reach of government into health care does not imply that market forces are a "cure all" for the many shortcomings of our current system. Without denying that managed care may be able to contribute to the solution, we must be wary of undue expectations. In order to improve our pluralistic health care system, which depends on both private and public sector dollars, we must reassess how each sector can interact with the other more effectively and efficiently.

By keeping this kind of matrix in mind, you will be able to follow the various debates and discussions covering the spectrum of health care reform that will continue over the next few years.

THE BUSINESS SIDE OF MEDICINE:
A Survival Primer for Medical Students and Residents

A State for Managed Competition

Managed competition may be defined as follows: A theory, originally proposed in 1993 by the Jackson Hole Group, that suggests that the individual employee receive a fixed sum from his or her employer. The individual employee chooses a health plan. If the plan chosen costs more than the employer's fixed sum, the employee is responsible for the difference. The individual employee would have a tax incentive to select lower priced options, because he or she would be able to deduct the amount of only the lowest cost option. The proposal's proponents believe this would encourage individual consumers of health care to be more price conscious. They also believe this will cause health care insurers to hold down the cost of their plans to make them more competitive.

The Florida approach to managed competition is illustrative of the concept. The Florida Plan does not include an employer mandate but rather is a voluntary program. In order to achieve cost containment, the plan has hospital rate setting and budget review, includes annual budget targets but not budget requirements, and has retained the certificate-of-need element. The key focus is insurance reform for small employers, including guaranteed renewal of insurance, portability of insurance between places of employment, and a move toward a modified "community rating"—that is, moving away from the current "experience rating" approach. Access and coverage are to be achieved through a system of 11 community health purchasing alliances (CHPAs) to pool the resources of small employers and also to include Medicaid.

The reason for putting together these CHPAs, especially focused on small employers, is that small businesses frequently do not offer health insurance as part of their benefit packages primarily because of cost. Florida has a high proportion of small businesses, some 36 percent or about 145,000 businesses, that do not offer health insurance coverage. Despite pessimistic predictions that the majority of small employers are not interested in offering health insurance as a benefit, irrespective of cost, early results show almost 80,000 workers and their dependents are covered, approximately 50 percent of whom were previously uninsured.

The state-created CHPAs have cost approximately $5 million dollars to establish. This is viewed as a positive outcome, because approximately 80 percent of those dollars, which otherwise would have been written off as charity care by community hospitals, now go directly to pay for health care. Bottom line is that a $5 million initial investment has generated almost $50 million in health care that otherwise would have been paid by the general public through taxes.

In addition, former Florida Governor Chiles was able to obtain a Medicaid waiver that permits the state to shift Medicaid recipients gradually into a variety of managed care programs. Despite disturbing evidence of fraud and abuse in the Medicaid Managed

Care Program, there has been enough real progress that the legislature has decided to shift Medicaid into two types of managed care programs: a primary care physician management program called MediPass and a traditional managed care program. Medicaid recipients in Florida will be divided between Medicaid and MediPass. It is believed that such a move will cost the state about 14 percent less than the current Medicaid program. At last count, of the approximately 1.5 million Medicaid eligibles, 250,000 are in MediPass, 413,000 are in managed care, and 828,000 remain in traditional fee-for-service Medicaid.

A significant number of health reform initiatives have been implemented at the state level. They run the gamut from the Florida Managed Care/Managed Competition Model, through play or pay approaches in Massachusetts, through prioritization of services in Oregon, to Hawaiian initiatives that are often pointed out as being ideal. (Hawaii has an employer mandate, plus community rating, and covers well over 95 percent of its population.) However, in the current political climate, it is obvious that not only is the federal government backing away from any major reform, but also the states are backing away from comprehensive reform. Two distinct and rapidly developing market strategies are evolving:

- Purchasing cooperatives (such as those in California, the Twin Cities, and Florida).

- Aggregation of providers and insurers into integrated delivery systems.

Health Insurance Portability and Accountability Act of 1996

The Kassebaum-Kennedy Bill allows for portability of insurance when people change employment by decreasing the pre-existing medical condition limitation to no more than two months. In addition, it decreases pre-existing condition limitation exclusions for up to one year. Exclusions based on health status for the offering of health insurance are prohibited. The bill also guarantees availability to the small group insurance market and renewability of coverage, regardless of health status of the individual. As mentioned earlier and discussed more fully below, the law offers a new experiment for Medicare called medical savings accounts and imposes some new and very heavy-handed fraud and abuse language.

The Kassebaum-Kennedy legislation will, for the first time at the federal level, launch an MSA experiment for a maximum of some 750,000 people, who will be allowed to participate in a four-year demonstration project (figure 9, page 20). The way in which medical savings accounts work is that individuals who participate in the program are allowed to establish tax deductible MSAs (very much like tax deductible IRAs) through contributions from their employers or through their own contributions. The individual

THE BUSINESS SIDE OF MEDICINE:

A Survival Primer for Medical Students and Residents

then has the ability to withdraw money from this tax-exempt MSA to pay for medical expenses. In addition, unused MSA funds can be accumulated and rolled forward into future years. MSAs must be coupled with high-deductible, no copayment, catastrophic health insurance plans, estimated to cost somewhere from $1,500 to $2,500 per year for an individual and from $3,000 to $4,500 a year for family coverage. MSA funds can be used for any medical expense currently deductible from federal income taxes, such as long-term care insurance, premiums for COBRA, as well as health care payments to physicians, hospitals, etc.

The theory is that patients under MSAs would feel very accountable for their health care, because, in a sense, they would be spending their own money, the MSA money. Two major concerns will be tested by this experiment:

- Such an approach might encourage people to avoid seeing doctors, thereby not getting necessary or appropriate care, especially preventive care, such as flu shots etc.

- The approach may be prone to adverse selection—that is, people who pick MSAs may be healthier, leaving sicker people to select traditional plans. The managed care plans would then fall into a higher risk pool. To theorists, this is a very exciting health reform experiment in returning responsibility and accountability for health care to individual patients.

Health Insurance Portability and Accountability Act of 1996

Provision	
Portability	Pre-existing condition limitation periods reduced with no more than a two-month break.
Pre-existing Condition Limitations	Allows imposition of exclusions for up to 12 months for physical or mental conditions diagnosed or treated within the previous six months.
Exclusions Based on Health Status	Prohibited.
Guaranteed Availability in Small Group Market	Requires insurers offering coverage to businesses with 2 to 50 employees to accept all small employers in that particular state, regardless of health status.
Guaranteed Renewability	Requires insurers offering group health coverage in the small or large group market to renew or continue coverage, regardless of health status.
Guaranteed Availability of Individual Coverage	Prohibits insurers from declining to offer coverage or denying enrollment to an individual who had group health insurance 18 or more months.
Guaranteed Renewal	Requires insurers to renew or continue individual coverage policy.
Medical Savings Accounts (MSAs)	Allows employees of small businesses (50 or fewer workers) and the self-employed to open tax-deductible MSAs in conjunction with high-deductible health plans, with a cap of 750,000 policies for four-year pilot project.
High-Risk Insurance Pools	Grants tax-exempt status to state-established, non-profit organizations providing health coverage to high-risk individuals.
Fraud and Abuse	Establishes national health care fraud and abuse control program; allows termination of Medicare HMO contract or intermediate sanctions for failing to carry out contract.
Health Insurance Premium Tax Deduction for Self-Employed	Increases incrementally from current 30% to 80% in 2006 and thereafter.
Long-Term Care Insurance and Services	Excludes reimbursements from income, treats premiums as medical expenses for tax purposes.

SOURCE: Washington Health Week

Figure 9

Since passage of the MSA rule, some 3,000 employers have offered MSAs, with some 35 insurers offering this option. Although this is not a major shift, there is growing interest in this new approach. More than 25,000 policies have been sold to date.

Despite the Kassebaum-Kennedy Bill, some very significant health care issues, such as Medicare and its predicted bankruptcy, remain. As a consequence, a very major and significant piece of legislation was passed to address a number of compelling issues. It is called the Balanced Budget Act of 1997. Both Democrats and Republicans proudly announced that they were able to agree to balance the budget sometime within the next five years.

Over the next five years, Congress projected a savings of more than $116 billion dollars. A significant portion of these dollars would come from hospital care, home care, skilled nursing facilities, and managed care. It is noteworthy that, although significant dollars are extracted from physician payments, they are very small compared to the other elements in the savings package.

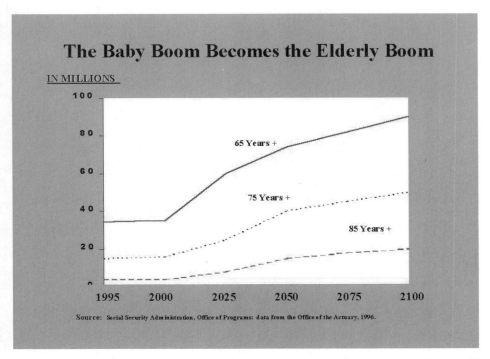

Figure 10

These areas were focused on by Congress because they were the major areas of Medicare spending increases in the recent past, especially hospital inpatient and home care. Medicare enrollment has been growing by leaps and bounds since 1974 and is estimated to more than double by the year 2015. As the "baby boomers" grow older, there will be a significant increase in the number of people who are 65 years or older. Of even greater significance is the major increase in the elderly—85 years of age and older as well as 75 years of age and older (figure 10, page 21). All of these demographic changes will stress the Medicare Program. It was strongly believed by all analysts that, if something were not done, the Part A Medicare Trust Fund would be bankrupt by the year 2001.

With enactment of the Balanced Budget Act of 1997, the following results are predicted. Instead of bankruptcy occurring when reserves from the Medicare Part A Trust Fund are exhausted in the year 2001, it is now projected that this will occur sometime after the year 2006, or perhaps even closer to the year 2010 (figure 11, below). Therefore, there has been a temporary defusion in anxiety about the bankruptcy of this key social program, although most individuals do not believe that the problem for the upcoming baby boomers is truly solved. For that reason, the President and the Congress have just appointed a top-level commission, the National Bipartisan Committee on the Future of

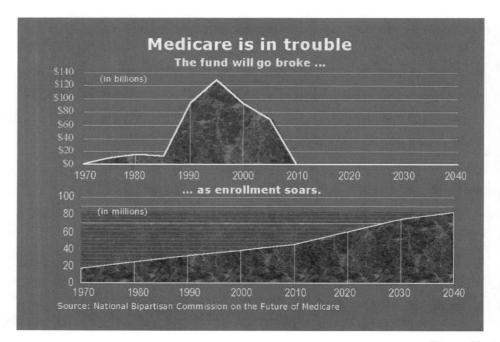

Figure 11

Medicare (also called the "Boomer Commission") to review the future direction of Medicare and to address its ultimate solvency.

What About Managed Care?

Managed care has been viewed by employers and government as a major strategy for addressing the increasing costs of health care. However, recently, and increasingly, there have been growing horror stories about managed care, wherein families are being stressed by managed care companies' decisions relative to treatment and are being forced to abandon long-term relationships with their physicians. There is growing publicity concerning "drive-through" mastectomies and deliveries, the highly publicized shift of managed care to the for-profit sector, and the related concern that Wall Street greed will diminish the resources necessary to provide high-quality health care to enrollees. These stories and concerns have prompted a variety of responses from health care plans and from providers, such as hospitals and physicians, both at the state legislature level and in Congress.

Numerous laws have been proposed at the state level. As these sometimes uncoordinated legislative pieces have been enacted, there has been growing concern that these well-intentioned but perhaps misguided interventions are "playing doctor" and will ultimately make a mess of things and run up costs. There is now an interest in creating a more umbrella-like legislative approach at the state and the federal levels.

This is especially evident in California, where the governor vetoed all managed care regulatory legislation to wait for the report of his oversight managed care commission. In addition, President Clinton appointed an Advisory Commission on Consumer Protection and Quality, charged with studying and making recommendations on managed care in specific and health care in general.

Finally, a significant new issue is the growing number of uninsured and the fact that these 43+ million people include 10+ million children. At both the federal and the state levels, this issue is being addressed in a variety of ways. Only time will tell how effective this approach will be.

Imbedded in the Balanced Budget Act of 1997 is an entire new section of Medicare called Medicare Plus Choice, also known as Medicare Part C. Medicare Part C offers new options for financing the care of Medicare recipients. In addition to traditional Medicare Part A and Part B, which follow the traditional indemnity approach, under Medicare Part C there will be:

- Further emphasis on Medicare risk contracts.

- Development of a concept called provider service organizations (PSOs).

- Further development of medical savings account options.

- A private fee-for-service plan.

The latter option permits Medicare beneficiaries to drop out of the standard Medicare program and enter into private contracts with physicians for selected services. In addition, it allows Medicare beneficiaries to enroll in private indemnity insurance plans, which would give them more latitude in selecting providers.

These changes raise very significant political issues. Some people predict it is the beginning of a shift to a two-class Medicare system and changes Medicare from what it currently is—a defined benefit plan—to what some individuals would like Medicare to be—a defined contribution plan or premium support model. Nonetheless, the Balanced Budget Act of 1997 was enacted, and HCFA is very busy developing regulations for implementing the various elements of the plan, including the new Medicare-C Options.

The health care reform debate addressing cost, access, and Medicare bankruptcy will continue and evolve. Only time can tell what types of specific approaches will be embraced. It is safe to predict, however, that the current tendency to address budgetary and fiscal issues will be a predominant focus in the near term.

It is becoming more and more evident that many people really believe that health care should not be just another commodity or product, but rather a social good, such as food and shelter and, therefore, should be dealt with in a highly professional manner. The difference is obvious—a commodity is usually just a commercial venture in which it is very appropriate to maximize profits. On our current trajectory, health care might not be handled in an appropriate and socially acceptable manner when we are dealing with managed care, capitation, employed physicians with withholds, and incentives that may well force physicians to be more concerned about their own economic well-being than, perhaps, the well-being of their patients. There is a growing sentiment that, ultimately, we may have to develop rules on how health care will operate so that the current industrialization and commercialization of medicine do not become too brutal and so that concerns about quality will not be lost.

References

1. *The World Medical Market Fact File 1997.* London, England: Market Line International, Dec. 1996.

2. Anderson, O. "Government Health Insurance and Privatization: An Examination of the Concept and of Equity." *International Journal of Health Planning and Management* 3(1):35-43, Jan.-Feb. 1988.

3. Blendon, R. "Who Has the Best Health Care System? A Second Look." *Health Affairs* 14(4):220-30, Winter 1995.

4. The Gallup Organization, The Gallup Building, 47 Hulfish Street, Princeton, N.J. 08542.

5. Hugh Scott, MD, Executive Director of the Royal College of Physicians and Surgeons, Canada. Personal communication, 1998.

CHAPTER 2

The Evolution of Managed Care

The basic concepts of managed care—capitation and integration—can be traced to the 1800s, to the funeral and benevolent societies that immigrants brought to this country in order to cover death expenses. Recruited to work in very isolated geographic areas, such as the sugar and pineapple plantations of Hawaii; lumber camps in Michigan, Wisconsin, and Washington; mines and iron ranges in northern Minnesota; and, of course, the railroads that proliferated throughout the country, the immigrants and their employers pioneered capitated health care and organized delivery of services patterned after those societies. Physicians were hired and placed on salary. They traveled with the companies, tending to the needs of accident victims and disabled workers.

The Mayo Clinic, founded by brothers William and Charles Mayo in 1883, became the first full-time, multispecialty group practice; as early as 1929, some 386 physicians and dentists were employed by the Mayo Clinic. The Mayo Clinic model became the prototype for multispecialty integration, which enabled grouped physicians to accept capitation and risk contracts.

Loosely modeled after the successful Mayo model, new health care organizations began springing up in the 1920s and 1930s, including the Elk City Cooperative and the Ross-Loos Clinic—the first capitated health plan. Kaiser Permanente, which is now the largest group-model HMO in existence, was formed in the 1940s.

Already strong, the managed care movement received national attention and legitimacy with passage of the Health Maintenance Organization Act of 1973. Paul Ellwood, MD, advisor to then-President Richard Nixon and a major influence in enactment of the Act, coined the term HMO.[1] The Act passed because of some of the same concerns facing this country today: rising Medicare and Medicaid costs. Its passage ignited the growth of managed care organizations.

The Force Behind Managed Care

Until very recently, American physicians and hospitals dominated the health care system clinically, economically, and politically. Provider dominance was fueled by a relatively passive third-party insurer system and the principle that all patients had the right to a free choice of providers. Under such a system of supply-side economics and fee-for-service medicine, combined with the autonomy of providers, especially physicians, it is not surprising that the size, configuration, and total cost of the American health system increased at double-digit rates, until, today, it consumes close to 14 percent of the Gross Domestic Product or approximately $1 trillion annually.

It was only a matter of time, therefore, until those who write the checks—employers, who account for some 35 percent of health care expenditures, and federal and state government, which account for nearly 44 percent of health care spending—became the driving forces for using managed care as the mechanism to control rising health care costs.

How Does Managed Care Control Costs?

In order to answer this question, it is helpful to look at health care expenditures from a different angle. Instead of looking at hospital care and physician services, we should look at the macroeconomic reasons for increasing costs.

The sources of health care cost increases can be divided into four major categories: general inflation, population increases, medical price inflation in excess of general inflation, and increases in the volume and the intensity of services.

If the objective is to control health care costs to the level of the per capita inflation rate, general price inflation and population changes are acceptable causes for increases. However, volume and intensity of services and excess medical price growth are unacceptable increases under such an objective. And they add up to nearly 50 percent of the problem.

The reasons for high growth in volume and intensity of services includes new technologies, more technologies per patient, aging of the population, focus on new diseases, etc. However, no matter how rational the reasons for increases in volume or intensity of services, managed care organizations are determined to control them and what they view as excessive increases in medical costs.

Health Care Delivery in the '70s

When providers had economic and political dominance over the American health system prior to the shift to managed care, the patient got insurance coverage through either an employer or the government, which passively paid premiums to an insurance company. The insurance company paid on a passive, fee-for-service basis to primary care physicians, specialty physicians, and hospitals (figure 1, page 29). As fee-for-service costs from hospitals, specialists, and primary care physicians rose, premiums to employers and/or government went up, but patients were insulated from the costs of health care services by the payer of the insurance—the government or the employer. As mentioned earlier, these changes have further fueled volume and intensity of services and stimulated excessive growth in medical costs. Total costs of U.S. health care have risen past $1 trillion a year and reached more than 14 percent of the country's Gross Domestic Product.

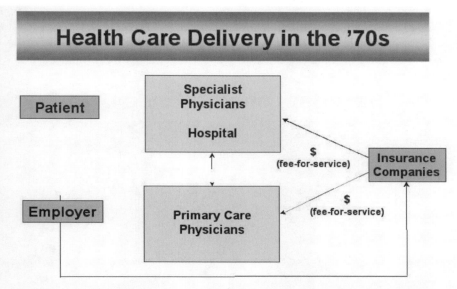

Figure 1

As a consequence of both business and government wishing to control controllable variables and health care costs, the financing of health care delivery was reformatted in the 1980s and early 1990s (figure 2, below). As recently as 1992, indemnity insurance made up 52 percent of the benefit packages employers offered to employees. However,

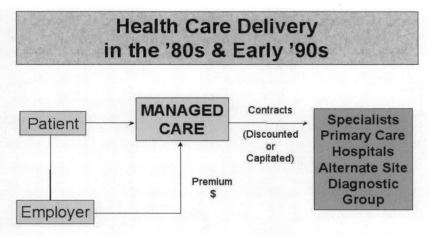

Figure 2

the figure decreased to 32 percent in 1994. It decreased to 18 percent in 1997, with the remaining 82 percent of benefits being offered through managed care (figure 3, below). Managed care companies now act as intermediaries between patients and employers. Employers or government pay most of the premiums to managed care companies.

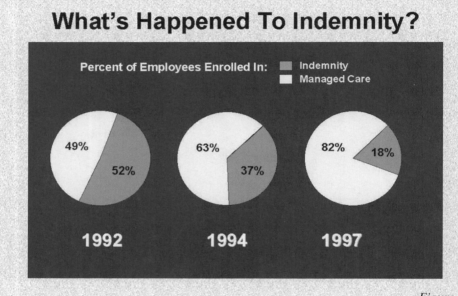

Figure 3

In the 1970s, 1980s, and even early 1990s, insurers acted as passive third parties. Now, insurers are active managers and players, not only in financing insurance but also in directing how, where, and by whom health services will be delivered. Called "selective contracting," the latter activities are the major mechanism by which control is shifted from the supply side to the demand side of the health sector equation. Insurers are empowered to limit insureds to a set of preferred providers and thus exclude any provider found by the health plan to be wanting for any reason—because prices are too high or resources used in treating illnesses exceed explicit guidelines. "Any Willing Provider" laws have been passed in a number of states in attempts to curtail the practice of selective contracting.

Four basic elements characterize the activities of managed care plans and are an extension of the economic leverage of selective contracting:

- They contract with providers to furnish comprehensive services to plan subscribers. These contracts establish what services will be provided and at what prices.

- They establish explicit standards for selecting providers. For physicians, managed care organizations utilize performance profiles, such as analysis of practice habits, outcomes measures, and patient satisfaction surveys. When looking at other providers, such as hospitals, they utilize gross measurements, such as accreditation, ranges of services, mortality rates, morbidity rates, and other data.

- Quality assurance and utilization management programs are the cornerstones and essential components of every managed care program. The goal of quality assurance and utilization management is to monitor the quality, necessity, and appropriateness of medical interventions.

- Financial incentives are put in place by managed care companies to encourage patients to use selected providers. They do this by requiring larger copayments when patients use providers outside the contracted network.

How Do Managed Care Companies Manage Costs?

Managed care organizations use treatment protocols and practice guidelines, drug formularies, and peer review to micromanage patient care within the four elements outlines above.

- Treatment protocols or practice guidelines are constructed from sound data and evidence-based medicine, but, like all guidelines, sometimes they do not take into consideration unique issues facing individual patients.

- Managed care companies mandate drug formularies that frequently require the use of generic drugs and limit the types of drugs that can be utilized for specific conditions.

- Frequently, they utilize peer review to determine "appropriate utilization." Through utilization management, managed care companies can require authorization for all referrals from one physician to another and preauthorization review of selected procedures, especially invasive procedures. Concurrent reviews are utilized during hospitalizations and usually are performed by nurses or other administrative personnel in the hospital.

There has been very significant growth in enrollment in managed care organizations since the early 1980s as a consequence of endorsement of this mechanism by employers and government (figure 4, page 32). It is predicted that, by the year 2000, HMOs and PPOs will control some 65 percent of the market, with managed fee-for-service and regular fee-for-service plans reduced to about 20 percent of the market.

Capitation

One of the primary fiscal mechanisms used by managed care organizations to control

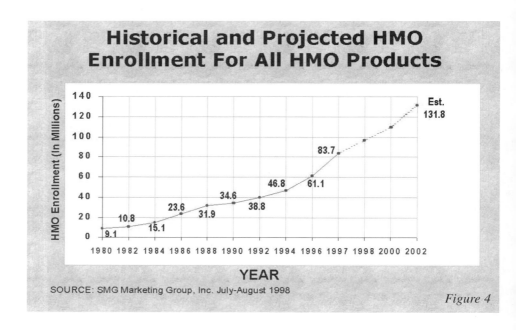

Figure 4

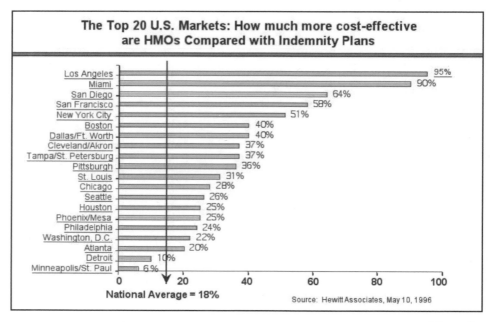

Figure 5

the market is called "capitation." Under capitation, a provider is paid a fixed fee for all services rendered over a specific period. It is usually referred to as payment per member per month (PMPM). Providers assume financial risk for costs that exceed capitation payments. They are thus given an incentive to provide only necessary and appropriate care. The insurer accepts the financial risk of illness for a population through the premium and then immediately shifts the risk to providers. This risk shifting is the essence of capitation.

In addition to shifting financial risk to providers, managed care results in significant savings. On average, managed care plans are 18 percent cheaper than traditional indemnity plans. The greatest variance between managed care and indemnity occurs in areas such as Los Angeles and Miami; it is less dramatic in areas such as Detroit and Minnesota (figure 5, page 32).

Markets go through four highly predictable evolutionary stages of managed care development (figure 6, below)—moving from unstructured in Stage I to managed competition in Stage IV. Figure 7, page 34, shows the managed care evolution for several U.S. cities. A number of areas remain relatively immune to the trend, but

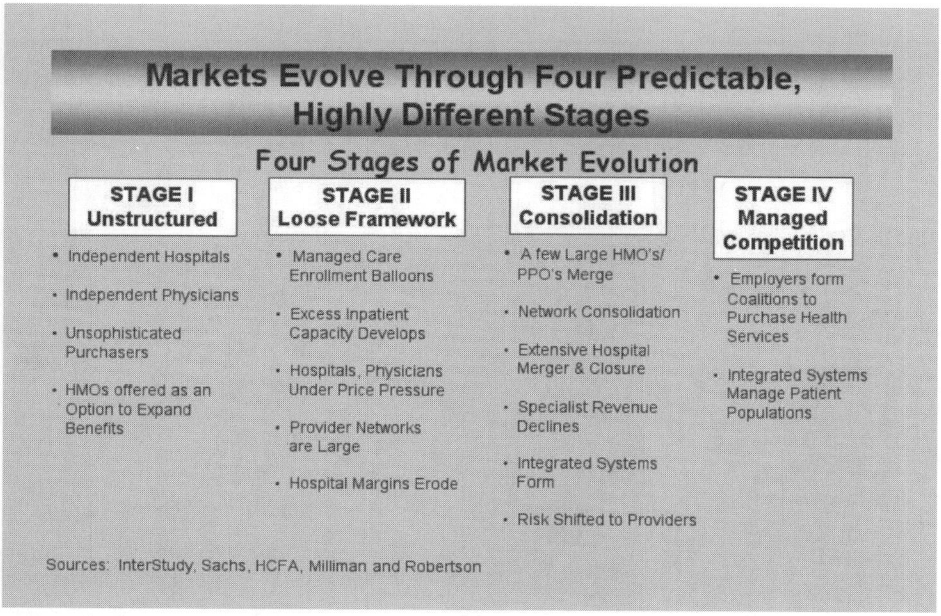

Markets Evolve Through Four Predictable, Highly Different Stages

Four Stages of Market Evolution

STAGE I Unstructured	STAGE II Loose Framework	STAGE III Consolidation	STAGE IV Managed Competition
• Independent Hospitals	• Managed Care Enrollment Balloons	• A few Large HMO's/ PPO's Merge	• Employers form Coalitions to Purchase Health Services
• Independent Physicians	• Excess Inpatient Capacity Develops	• Network Consolidation	
• Unsophisticated Purchasers	• Hospitals, Physicians Under Price Pressure	• Extensive Hospital Merger & Closure	• Integrated Systems Manage Patient Populations
• HMOs offered as an Option to Expand Benefits	• Provider Networks are Large	• Specialist Revenue Declines	
	• Hospital Margins Erode	• Integrated Systems Form	
		• Risk Shifted to Providers	

Sources: InterStudy, Sachs, HCFA, Milliman and Robertson

Figure 6

increasing numbers have arrived at Stage III—consolidation.

Has managed care significantly decreased employers' health care costs? As shown in figure 8, page 35, the effect has been dramatic. One does not have to be an economics genius to understand why employers are pleased and why managed care is growing rapidly. As a consequence of the major shift to managed care, and of a general decline in inflation in the U.S. economy, percentage increases in health care costs have fallen from the 15-20 percent levels of the late 1980s and early 1990s to very modest levels in recent years (figure 9, page 35). Although some upward creep in the increases is anticipated, double-digit increases seem unlikely.

Managed care's achievements on the government's side have been just as dramatic. According to a study done by the American Association of Health Plans and Price Waterhouse in 1996,[2] comparing Medicare average costs per month for HMO members with costs for fee-for-service patients, fee-for-service costs are significantly higher than those for managed care. In addition, when what current Medicare HMO members would pay if they switched to fee-for-service is calculated, the variance is even more significant. These kinds of data are certain to influence the federal government to accelerate the shift toward use of managed care.

1996 Market Evolution Model

Stage 1 Unstructured		Stage 2 Loose Framework		Stage 3 Consolidation		Stage 4 Hypercompetitive	
Knoxville, TN	1.5	Gainesville, FL	2.0	Salt Lake City, UT	2.9	Sacramento, CA	3.5
Middlesex, NJ	1.5	Harrisburg, PA	2.0	Milwaukee, WI	2.8	Minneapolis/St. Paul, MI	3.5
Augusta, GA	1.5	Lexington, KY	2.0	Denver, CO	2.7	Portland, OR	3.4
Charleston, SC	1.5	Pittsburgh, PA	2.0	Worcester, MA	2.5	Los Angeles, CA	3.3
Iowa City, IA	1.5	Indianapolis, IN	1.9	Baltimore, MD.	2.5	San Diego, CA	3.3
Mobile, AL	1.5	Nashville, TN	1.9	Memphis, TN	2.5	San Jose, CA	3.3
Shreveport, LA	1.5	New York, NY	1.8	Cincinnati, OH	2.4	San Francisco, CA	3.2
Charlottesville, VA	1.4	New Haven, CT	1.8	Seattle, WA	2.4	Orange County, CA	3.2
Little Rock, AR	1.4	Hartford, CT	1.8	Albany, NY	2.3	Madison, WI	3.0
Morgantown, WV	1.4	Syracuse, NY	1.8	Boston, MA	2.3	Tucson, AZ	3.0
Columbia, MO	1.3	Nassau-Suffolk, NY	1.7	Cleveland, OH	2.3		
Greenville, NC	1.2	Newark, NJ	1.7	Kansas City, MO	2.2		
		Birmingham, AL	1.6	Chicago, IL	2.2		
		Omaha, NE-IA	1.6	Philadelphia, PA	2.2		
		Chapel Hill, NC	1.6	Richmond, VA	2.2		
		Galveston, TX	1.5	St. Louis, MO	2.2		
		Winston-Salem, NC	1.5	Houston, TX	2.2		
				Atlanta, GA	2.2		
				Columbus, OH	2.2		
				Toledo, OH	2.2		
				Washington, DC	2.2		
				Ann Harbor, MI	2.1		
				Oklahoma City, OK	2.1		
				Dallas, TX	2.1		

Source: InterstudySachs, HCFA Milliman and Robertson

© University Health System Consortium

Figure 7

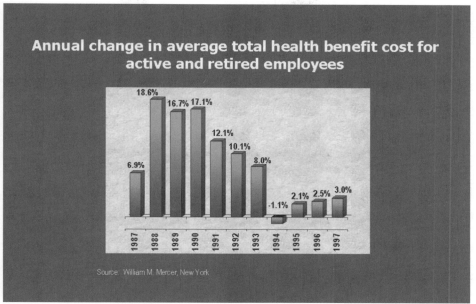

Figure 8

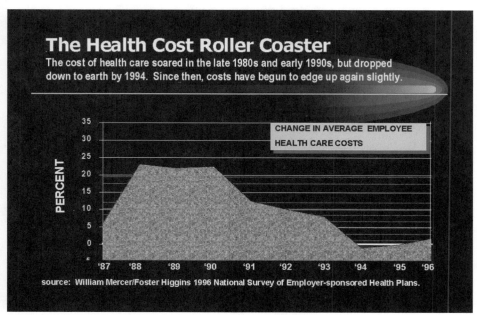

Figure 9

From a modest beginning just a decade ago, the Medicare managed care population had grown to 5 million elderly by the end of 1997. The number of enrollees is expected to reach 15 million by 2007, which would represent about one-third of all Medicare beneficiaries (figure 10, below).

A real question arises over whether Medicare-eligible individuals are content with their managed care coverage. All evidence to date suggests that the vast majority of Medicare beneficiaries are satisfied with managed care coverage. Examples of dissatisfaction exist, but those who move from managed care plans normally select other such plans. A 1998 survey confirmed early HCFA studies that found that the majority of Medicare HMO enrollees indicate satisfaction with their plans and have high satisfaction with the quality of care provided by their primary care physicians and specialists.[3]

Medicaid Managed Care

In the past few years, a number of states—Arizona, Oregon, Pennsylvania, and Tennessee, for instance—have received Medicaid waivers that have enabled them to shift their Medicaid populations into managed care. Currently, nearly 50 percent of the eligible Medicaid population is in managed care plans (figure 11, page 37).

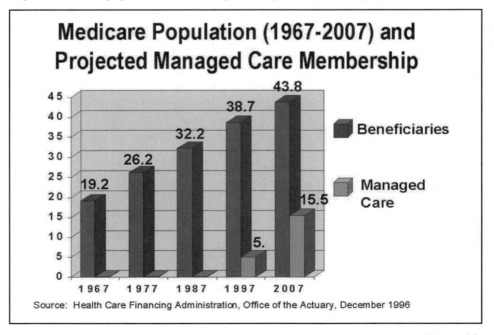

Source: Health Care Financing Administration, Office of the Actuary, December 1996

Figure 10

It is informative to look at exactly how the premium dollar is allocated by a managed care organization. Of the 100 percent contributed by payers, some percentage—say 3 percent—is put aside as retained earnings or profit. Another percentage—say 6 percent—is used for third-party administration costs, and yet another—say 9 percent— for integrated delivery system or medical staff organization administration. That leaves 82 percent of the premium for medical care, of which 5 percent is put aside in a risk pool for providers. This reserve exists in case medical care expenditures are greater than the 77 percent of premium allocated for medical services. If costs exceed 77 percent, they are covered from the risk pool. If costs are less, the risk pool is distributed as a bonus from primary care physician funds, specialty funds, hospital funds, and ancillary services funds.

Most of the growth in managed care organizations over the past five years has occurred in the for-profit sector, so that today they constitute more than 50 percent of the market. This shift to the for-profit sector should be and is a great cause of concern to providers, because inherent in for-profit ventures is a requirement of a return-on-investment, which ultimately must come at the expense of patient care services.

The business community takes the position that there is nothing illegal or immoral in an

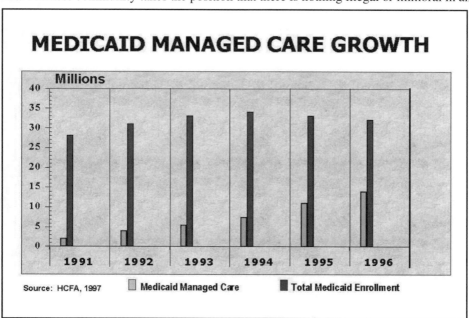

MEDICAID MANAGED CARE GROWTH

Source: HCFA, 1997   ☐ Medicaid Managed Care   ■ Total Medicaid Enrollment

Figure 11

industry making a profit. In fact, if the industry did not make a profit, there would be no industry. In health care, on the other hand, we have had a tradition of community-based, not-for-profit organizations. The profit in these organizations—i.e., the difference between income and expenses—has traditionally been returned to the community in some way, either by increasing services to the community or by modernizing facilities. In the for-profit Wall Street sector, profits are distributed to stockholders and are, therefore, not re-invested in the local community.

While the jury is still out on the success of managed care's cost control and medical micromanagement and on whether managed care companies are really effecting what they are supposed to effect, there is growing evidence that managed care can indeed reap substantial savings without affecting quality. Lower health care costs do not necessarily translate into inferior health care results. Many studies have demonstrated that, in geographic areas with significant penetration of managed care (figure 12, below), there are significantly lower costs and reduced hospital lengths of stay. Mortality rates have also been shown to be lower under managed care.

The criticism of a few years ago that managed care attracted primarily patients who were less sick and could save money from one-time events has been overridden by more recent data. It is now evident that managed care plans are just as likely as indemnity plans to have chronically ill patients and that, overall, managed care members are very similar to the fee-for-service population.

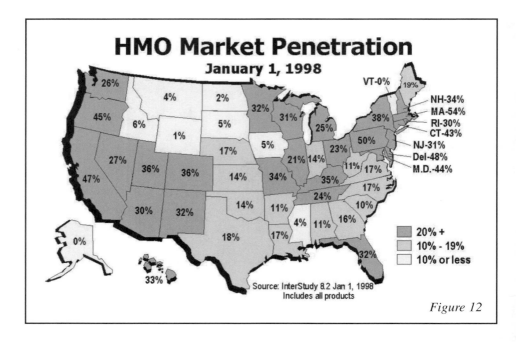

Figure 12

The Future of Managed Care

Managed care now enrolls some 80 million people, or almost 25 percent of the U.S. population, and grew in 1997 by some 20 million people. Although growth has not been equally distributed among the states, just about every state has seen some activity. California, Pennsylvania, New Jersey, Florida, and New York account for 45 percent of managed care enrollment gains.

All evidence points to continued growth of managed care, stimulated both from the employment-based insurance sector and from government through Medicaid and Medicare. With this growth, there will be continued widespread adoption of the utilization management techniques earlier noted, development of computerized networks of physician profiles, and development of financial and medical criteria for utilization review and physician credentialing.

In 1998, a significant percentage of managed care plans developed financial difficulty, with as many as one-half of the nation's 650 HMOs predicted to have lost money (figure 13, below). As a consequence, it is projected that HMOs will try to impose premium increases at a level of eight to 10 percent and focus on new open-access and point-of-service products. But those attempts will be resisted by major employers that have not felt that they have to respond to price increases.

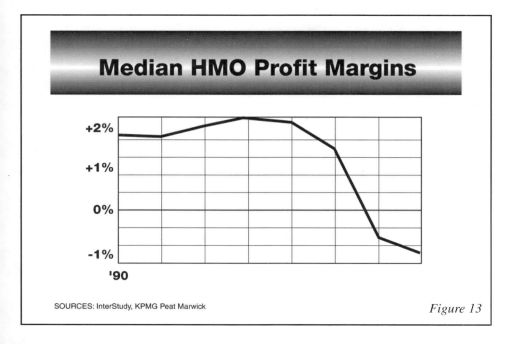

SOURCES: InterStudy, KPMG Peat Marwick

Figure 13

Like hospitals, which are experiencing decreasing occupancy and significantly lower lengths of stay, specialists are on the endangered species list in high-growth managed care areas. Only a small percentage of existing specialists in these markets are needed to serve enrollees. Managed care organizations delete these physicians from provider panels if their utilization and cost profiles are too high. On the other hand, "good performers" are increasingly being singled out for specialty network subcapitation or "carve-outs." In the beginning, specialists are paid on a discounted fee-for-service basis. At that point, all specialists can be included. Inevitably, however, as enrollment builds and costs rise, managed care plans develop data about "good performance" and identify specific groups of specialists for carve-outs. Many predict that use of the carve-out, sucapitation technique will accelerate. As a consequence of this changing environment, an increasing number of specialists are beginning to recognize that their future is best secured in a group configuration.

While you would think specialists would be a very unhappy lot, a recent survey of internal medicine specialists who are members of the American College of Physicians revealed that 57 percent of the membership said they were either somewhat satisfied or very satisfied with managed care. Forty-one percent were not satisfied.

Conclusions

So, what does the future seem to hold?

- Despite negative publicity, legislative actions, and generalized public angst, the health care system will continue to change, fueled primarily by managed care. Medicare and Medicaid reform will continue to present opportunities for growth for managed care organizations.

- Strong managed care organizations will continue to prosper as patients migrate from indemnity plans to managed care.

- Managed care organizations will return to profitability by increasing premiums and changing product lines, especially by introducing more open access and point of service options.

References

1. Ellwood, P. "Health Maintenance Organizations. Concept and Strategy." *Hospitals* 45(6):53-6, March 16, 1971.

2. Washington, D.C.: American Association of Health Plans, 1996.

3. *Survey of Medicare HMO Enrollees April-July 1998*. Chicago, Ill.: Towers Perrin, 1998.

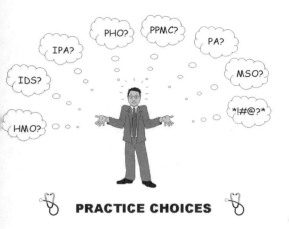

PRACTICE CHOICES

CHAPTER 3

The Medical Marketplace and Practice Consolidation

For the past 200 years, with a few rare exceptions, physicians have enjoyed total autonomy relative to their practices. They practiced solo, or in two- or three-person, single-specialty groups, until the late 1980s. Solo-practice, fee-for-service medicine was the unchallenged gold standard. Patients had the absolute right to select their health care providers, and solo-practice, fee-for-service medicine offered patients the best opportunity for ethical, high-quality medical care. Consequently, many physicians believe to this day that fee-for-service payment and solo practice offer better medical care than any other configuration.

Historical Characteristics of Physicians

Physicians have always preferred to work alone, to relate to patients on a one-on-one basis, and to have total freedom to select for their patients whatever medical interventions they feel are necessary, with very little regulatory oversight. In addition, they sought and usually achieved the authority and the freedom to regulate themselves.

Physicians can be generally characterized as doers, seeing a problem and acting on it, rather than as long-term strategists. And they are frequently characterized as having a very short-term orientation and looking for immediate gratification. Physicians are more interested, for example, in acute care interventional medicine than in preventive medicine and the care of populations.

Physicians view themselves as professionals, in all regards, and are deeply embedded in evidence-based practice that achieves high ethical and moral standards.

These traditional characteristics tend to make physicians somewhat reactionary and resistant to change. In fact, it has been suggested that most physicians "fear change more than disaster." As a consequence of the above-noted characteristics, they are often distrustful of others, take things personally, feel they have unlimited expertise, and are very concerned over equity issues. Physicians are frequently so self-reliant that they do not readily accept leadership from others.

Since 1950, the number of practicing U.S. physicians has significantly increased, from approximately 150 physicians per 100,000 to a projected 300 physicians per 100,000 by the year 2020, if nothing is done to modify the pipeline. Weiner, in what is perhaps the definitive recent study relative to the physician work force,[1] stated that, from his data, there is currently a surplus of 165,000 physicians, or 50 physicians per 100,000, and that this surplus lies primarily in the specialist ranks, with a primary care physician equilibrium. In recent years, a significant proportion of the increase in the physician workforce has been a consequence of a major influx of international medical graduates (IMGs), almost doubling between 1980 and 1994 (figure 1, below). The vast majority of IMGs trained in the United States remain to practice here.

Fee-for-service utilizes approximately 207 physicians per 100,000 population, whereas managed care utilizes only 120 physicians per 100,000. Evaluating these data and a number of other studies, conventional wisdom, at this point, is that there is currently an excess of physicians in the workplace, moving rapidly toward a true physician glut.

Physician Net Income

From 1985 to 1993, there was a steady and progressive increase in physician net income (figure 2, page 43). In 1994, for the first time ever, there was a dip. Physician income rebounded slightly in 1995 and 1996, but it is projected to either level off or dip further

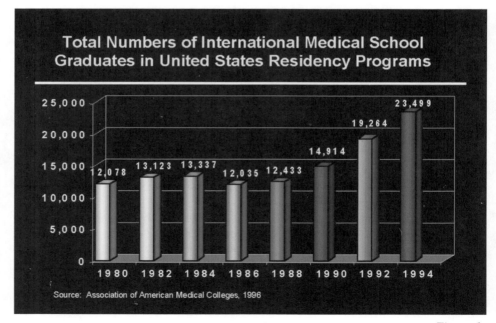

Figure 1

in the future. From an economic point of view, the market is beginning to speak, and physicians are beginning to be concerned about their incomes. Recent studies have demonstrated that the only way physicians have been able to maintain their incomes has been to significantly increase their productivity, because compensation for individual patient services has gone down significantly and is predicted to go down even further.

This trend can be readily understood by looking at Medicare payments over the past few years. There was a decrease in compensation for all specialties from Medicare between 1992 and 1996 that significantly affected specialists (figure 3, page 44). In addition, as a consequence of a shift to a single conversion factor in January 1998, further impacts of compensation from Medicare income are being felt. Office-based physicians, such as family practice physicians, dermatologists, and podiatrists, are doing well, while specialists are again being the hardest hit, especially cardiac surgeons, gasteroenterologists, etc.

Physicians, in a reaction to these negative forces, are looking at the following strategies to maintain their income levels:

• Downsizing office staff and standardizing supplies.

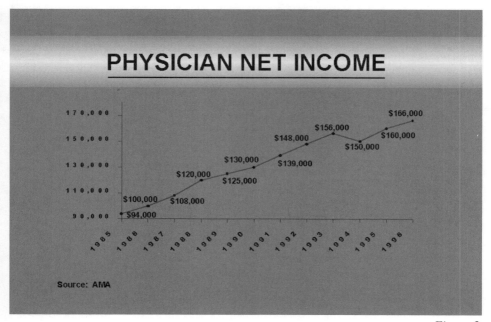

Figure 2

- Attempting to increase practice revenues by improving their coding policies; extending offices hours, opening satellite clinics, insourcing ancillary services, increasing patient visits per hour, and expanding their marketing efforts.

- Altering their practices—that is, exploring merger with other groups and/or entertaining for-profit offers.

Physician Unions

Physicians in some markets are looking to organized labor to help them combat these market forces. The Federation of Physicians and Dentists, an affiliate of AFL-CIO, is one of the more prominent union-organizing efforts, especially in Connecticut, Ohio, and Florida. The Florida-based union, which claims close to 8,000 members nationally, has been active in organizing orthopedists, neurosurgeons, obstetricians, and otolaryngologists. It has caught the attention of a significant number of physicians, despite the fact that this concept would have been antithetical to most physicians a few years ago. This particular union, however, has recently come under federal antitrust investigation for allegedly boycotting a managed care plan.

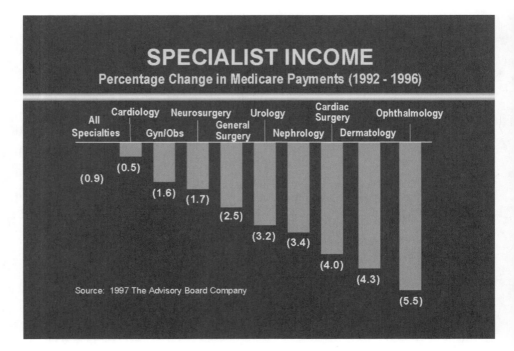

Figure 3

Interest in unionization has been particularly prominent among hospital-employed physicians. Examples are St. Barnabas Hospital in New York City, a 190-member physician group; Medalia Healthcare in Seattle, with 210 primary care physicians; and Rockford Illinois Health System, with a 170-physician multispecialty group. The impetus, physicians say, is that hospital administration implemented changes that affected them and patient care without seeking their input.

There is also a strong move among house staff members to unionize, especially in the Boston area. The Association of American Medical Colleges and the Liaison Commission on Medical Education have taken the position that house staff members are not employees and should not, therefore, have access to collective bargaining. Rather, they are students in an educational setting under the supervision of faculty. Many house staff groups are adamant that, as a result of managed care and the reduced numbers of house staff members, collective bargaining is necessary, and the effort is gathering momentum. The American Medical Association has not taken a stand one way or the other, but the National Labor Relations Board will soon take up the case.

Market forces pushing the shift from the supply side to the demand side and away from government regulation into the marketplace are obviously transforming the body and soul of American medicine. The key element enabling purchasers to force change on physicians and hospitals is the excess capacity of these elements in most health care markets.

One of the consequences of the move to the marketplace has been "merger mania." Hardly a day goes by without notice of some major merger or takeover in health care, especially in the hospital sector. Why this push toward mergers? The hope is that the consolidated organization will be more successful than single, autonomous organizations in eliminating duplicative and redundant facilities, equipment, and personnel and, thereby, will save money. In addition, consolidations not only are motivated by the search for efficiency but also are a tool to achieve increasing market power, power that can force lower prices for everything the organization buys and higher prices for what it sells. In other words, there is a desire to return leverage to the supply side of the equation.

The Rise of Vertically Integrated Systems

As a consequence of consolidation between 1994 and 1996, the number of vertically integrated health systems has increased from approximately 255 to more than 566. In areas with more integrated systems, the average cost per discharge has risen; where there is less integration—such as in Washington, D.C.; Baltimore, Maryland; and Riverside, California, with less than 40 percent of health care delivery in systems—costs per discharge are almost $1,000 less.

If you examine statistics between 1993 and 1996, you find that average U.S. hospital operating margins have peaked, so that individual hospitals have about a 5 percent operating margin, whereas major integrated systems have only a 2.5 percent operating margin. The bottom line is that, although the theory was good, at least up to now, creating major large hospital integrated systems has not resulted in economies of scale, deeper market penetration, or lower costs.

It was only a matter of time before those that write the checks—that is, government, which accounts for some 45 percent of all health care spending, and private employers, which paid 35 percent—reacted sharply to the rapid growth in health spending and began to develop enough political will to challenge the autonomy of physicians. The first attack came not from employers, but from the Medicare program.

In 1983, Medicare replaced traditional retrospective, cost-plus reimbursement to hospitals with the DRG payment approach. It was the first real attempt to shift a significant portion of the financial risk of a patient's hospitalization directly to those responsible for the patient's care: hospitals and physicians in those hospitals.

Then, in 1992, the federal government attacked the physician payment mechanism and implemented the Resource-Based Relative Value Scale (RBRVS), a system that related physician payments to medical work, practice expense, and malpractice expenses. In

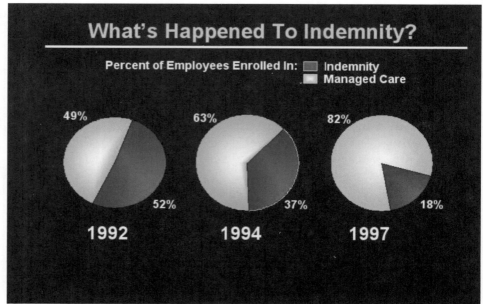

Figure 4

addition, conversion factors were implemented to more closely equalize surgical services, primary care services, and other nonsurgical services. As a consequence of the conversion factors, there were significant decreases in payments, especially to specialists, and some modest increases in payments to office-based primary care practitioners. This change reflected the leverage offered by an excess capacity of specialists in the marketplace.

As noted, after WW II, the primary vehicle for individuals to obtain health insurance was through their employment status. And, because of the favorable tax status of both employer and employee contributions, this benefit became more and more popular and grew, increasing to in excess of 25 percent of the total benefit costs of most employers. Employers began to look for remedies to the rapidly rising costs of their health care benefits and, not having the regulatory authority of government to enact things through the Health Care Financing Administration, have turned to managed care as the primary mechanism to control their costs.

What Happened to Indemnity?

In 1992, indemnity insurance comprised 52 percent of the health care benefit packages employers offered their employees. However, this decreased to 32 percent in 1994 and, in 1997, to 18 percent, with the remaining 82 percent of the benefit offered through the mechanism of managed care (figure 4, page 44). When private employers, anxious about the rising cost of health care, were able to persuade their employees to give up some freedom of choice of providers in return for continuing provision of employer-provided health insurance, it enabled them to shift to managed care and resulted in the rapid demise of the indemnity/fee-for-service mechanism of paying physicians. In managed care, diminished choice of providers is implemented through the mechanism of "selective contracting." Selective contracting is the vehicle utilized by managed care companies to dramatically move control from the supply side of the equation to the demand side of the equation. Selective contracting is the health plan's lever to limit the insured to a set of preferred providers. It gives the power to exclude any provider, either because the provider's prices are too high and/or, in the case of physicians, because the volume of treatments being applied to an individual patient exceeds an actuarially established clinical benchmark. Selective contracting has become the foundation of what we now refer to as "managed care."

Historical and Projected Enrollment for All HMO Products

HMO enrollment has risen rapidly, from fewer than 10 million enrollees in 1980 to 83 million enrollees in 1997. Enrollment is projected to pass 130 million by the year 2002 (figure 5, below). Has this shift to managed care achieved the cost savings employers seek?

The answer is a resounding yes. On average, national savings have been approximately 18 percent. In heavily penetrated managed care markets, the savings have been even more dramatic. For example, savings of 95 percent were achieved in Los Angeles, and Miami realized savings of 90 percent over indemnity plans.

The change in costs to employers has gone from double-digit changes in the mid-1980s to 2-3 percent increases in 1995, 1996, and 1997. Employers have definitely achieved their cost control goal by switching to managed care.

Since 1994, HMO profit margins have been going down (figure 6, page 49). In 1996, and through the third quarter of 1997, HMO profits disappear. Median HMO profit margins were down 1.2 percent in 1998, according to national accounting firm KPMG Peat Marwick. These trends have prompted analysts to predict that premiums will begin to rise. However, those predictions have not come to fruition yet, which may mean that there will be significant employer resistance to increasing premiums at this time.

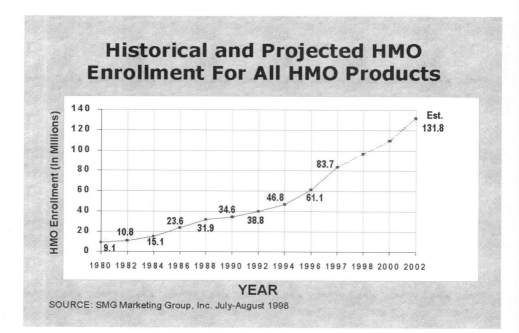

Figure 5

Health Care Delivery in the 1980s and the Early 1990s

There has been an effective shift of control from the supply side to the demand side and from government regulation to market forces. Today, the central focus is managed care, with patients; employers; and, more and more now, government seeking health care through the managed care mechanism. The premium goes to the managed care company that selectively contracts through discounts and/or capitated approaches to the supply side of the equation—specialists, primary care, hospitals, etc.

In low managed care penetration markets, physicians are still busy as ever. Indemnity continues to prevail, and fee for service is still the major mechanism of compensation for physicians. In medium managed care penetration markets, physicians are beginning to see the handwriting on the wall and are beginning to get organized into a variety of

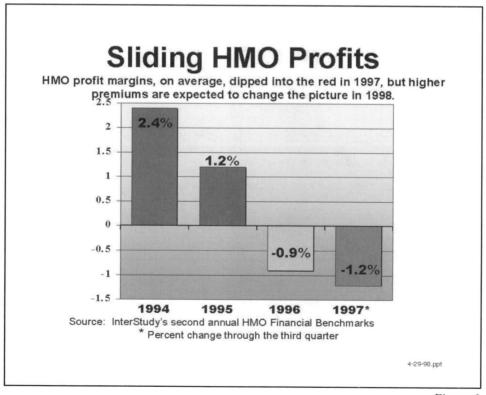

Figure 6

aggregations, such as PHOs, IPAs, etc. In highly penetrated markets, where risk arrangements are the prevailing mechanism, physician deselection is occurring, with very narrow provider panels but with some direct access to specialists and significant price pressures on both HMOs and providers being applied by government and business.

The number of group practices was very small in 1965 and gradually increased until 1984. It remained quite flat from 1984 to 1991, then spurted between 1991 and 1995. Another way of looking at these data is the percentage of physicians in group practice (figure 7, below). From a relatively minor percentage, 10 percent in 1965, groups gradually but progressively increased to almost 35 percent of physicians by 1995.

Yet another way of looking at these statistics is that the growth in group practice and the growth in employed physicians occurred at the expense of solo practice. As the market has shifted from the supply side to the demand side, physicians initially reacted by moving into group practice configurations and into employed relationships with a variety of institutions.

Therefore, in broad generalities, physicians are looking at options such as "toughing it out" in independent practice, an option most seriously considered by individuals closer

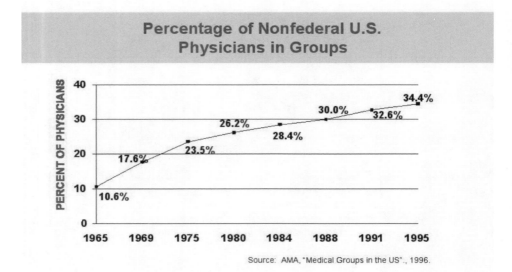

Source: AMA, "Medical Groups in the US"., 1996.

Figure 7

to the end of their professional careers; aggregating into a variety of group configurations; or becoming salaried employees. The latter two options are more attractive to younger, more recent graduates looking to employment opportunities rather than seeking to establish solo practices.

Health Care Organizations and Integrated Systems Rising

Between 1994 and 1996, there was a significant increase in consolidation and aggregation into integrated delivery systems, with some 38 percent of hospitals aggregating and managed care plans and physician clinics also aggregating (figure 8, below).

The key construct in the marketplace, therefore, has been one of merger and consolidation as managed care companies continue to consolidate, hospitals continue to merge and consolidate into larger systems, and physicians continue to form or join groups. All are seeking to create market power based on concentration of ownership and control in order to create a positive negotiating position relative to managed care. In

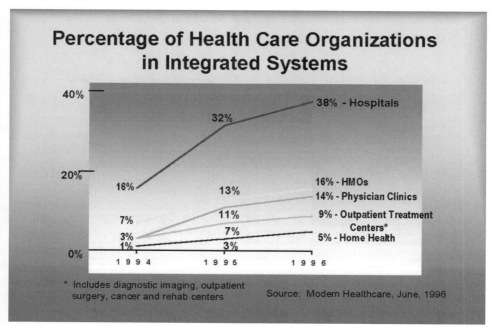

Percentage of Health Care Organizations in Integrated Systems

- 40%
- 38% - Hospitals
- 32%
- 20%
- 16% - HMOs
- 16%
- 14% - Physician Clinics
- 13%
- 11%
- 9% - Outpatient Treatment Centers*
- 7%
- 7%
- 5% - Home Health
- 3%
- 3%
- 1%
- 0%
- 1 9 9 4
- 1 9 9 5
- 1 9 9 6

* Includes diagnostic imaging, outpatient surgery, cancer and rehab centers

Source: Modern Healthcare, June, 1996

Figure 8

theory, the more beds and physicians in a health system, the more leverage that system has, because power in the current environment ultimately is derived from an ability to cut prices, increase market share, and spread costs over a larger base of operations.

In a very broad survey, managed care executives and for-profit and not-for-profit integrated systems were queried about how to achieve physician integration. The basic questions asked of them were what method was used and how effective the process has been (figure 9, below).[2] Medical service organizations (MSOs) are the most prominent method used to achieve physician organization, but they have only been 11 percent effective. The next most prominent method of integration, however, has been direct physician employment, which has been 44 percent effective, followed by PHOs, which have been only 19 percent effective. Practice management companies have penetrated some 51 percent, but were only 11 percent effective; closed PHOs were 40 percent used and only 14 percent effective.

Although aligning with physicians is a major methodology used in system integration, it

Models in Use to Increase Physician Integration, and Respondents Identifying Models as Most Effective

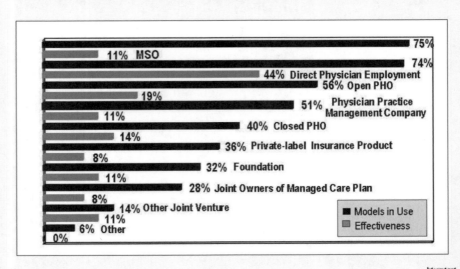

integrat.ppt

Figure 9

is the most difficult aspect of building an integrated delivery system. Physicians are very difficult to align, as discussed earlier. As a result, physicians in various markets are exploring formation of a variety of types of provider networks, including the following broad types of models.

IPA MODEL

The independent practice association (IPA) model is a very loose model wherein physicians, both primary care and specialists, form a new company. For purposes other than managed care, the individual physician practices often continue to remain autonomous; these physicians, not infrequently, link up with competing IPAs. More developed IPAs take on some administrative functions, such as marketing; contract management; information services; and, occasionally, billing and collecting. The advantages of an IPA are that it is simple to organize, is very flexible, and does not require much up-front capitalization. However, IPAs have some very significant problems:

- They do not generate any significant savings, because the practices are not tightly integrated.

- These linkages can raise a number of self-referral and kick-back questions under both federal (Stark) and state anti-self-referral legislation.

- IPAs can, if large enough, be subject to antitrust investigation relative primarily to price fixing and boycotting.

PHOs

The typical physician hospital organization (PHO) is a joint venture between physicians and a hospital. In its most simplistic form, the physician component can often be a loose IPA of physicians on the hospital staff. The hospital component of the PHO is not infrequently a for-profit subsidiary of the hospital. The for-profit mechanism is used because not-for-profit PHOs have a limitation restricting physician membership. Not infrequently, the PHO utilizes the hospital-based MSO organization to provide administrative services to the physicians and the PHO.

PHOs have had, at best, mixed reviews, either in reality or in perception. The hospital appears to be the dominant partner; controlling costs through the loose IPA has often been unsuccessful.

Hospital-Affiliated Medical Practices

A more advanced version of the PHO model occurs when the hospital sponsors a captive medical group. One of the common methodologies is when the hospital purchases the assets of physician practices and hires the physicians as employees. The physicians are then organized into a separate hospital-owned physician company. This model is more manageable than the simplistic PHO, because the hospital can impose control and discipline on the physician practices. The physicians also have a short-term gain from the sale of their practices.

In an even more sophisticated variation of the PHO, the hospital finances the creation of semi-autonomous medical groups, and contracts tight linkages between the hospital system and the captive medical groups and MSO services.

Between 1993 and 1995, these mechanisms of hospital-affiliated medical practices were a major trend. In 1993, some 4,000 physician practices were owned or managed by hospitals; by 1995, the number had increased to about 11,000, a 172 percent increase. Although there are no data beyond 1995, it is believed that growth has continued to a total of about 15,000 physician practices owned or managed by hospitals.

The vast majority of hospitals that have acquired physician practices are losing money; only about 15 percent are making money. Regardless, hospitals are still the most significant purchasers of physician practices, with physician practice management companies (PPMCs) and others making up less than 25 percent of the total.

Therefore, although there are exceptions, the general consensus, from a variety of studies, is that hospitals buying physician practices are, in the majority of cases, financial disasters. The consulting firm Coopers and Lybrand (now merged with Price Waterhouse to form PricewaterhouseCoopers) demonstrated that, on average, hospitals lose between $55,000 and $97,000 per physician/per year after buying a practice. The bottom line in 1997 was that the purchase of physician practices by hospitals might very well have been an error in business judgment.

Group Practice Model

The large, integrated, multispecialty group practice model was pioneered by Mayo Clinic, Cleveland Clinic, Ochsner Clinic, etc. This model is fully physician-directed and governed and has many advantages relative to federal and state anti-kickback and anti-self-referral laws. The model appears to be beneficial in terms of physician control and economies of scale. One of the problems in this model's growth has been raising capital, because capital needs must be met by contributions from individual physician owners, either directly or through borrowing. However, major law firms, accounting firms, and other professional service firms have financed themselves in this way for decades.

Investor Model

The capital needs just noted have stimulated the creation of the investor model, often referred to as the physician practice management company (PPMC). Here, the group practice, in effect, spins off all nonphysician services and administrative personnel into an entity that serves as an MSO, while the physicians and ancillary services remain in the previous organization. In return for spinning off the assets into the MSO corporation, the physicians receive cash and/or stock. The investors also can purchase stock in the MSO corporation and are, thereby, insulated from state laws relative to the practice of medicine.

However, a major hiccup occurred in Florida. In November 1997, the Florida Board of Medicine stated that it was illegal to pay a physician practice management company a performance-based fee if the company:

- Creates a physician provider network.

- Develops relationships and affiliations with other physician provider networks.

- Develops and provides ancillary services—including pharmacy, laboratory, and diagnostic services—or evaluates, negotiates, and administers managed care contracts.

The Board declared such actions "fee splitting" under Florida law. Such an action may well be grounds for disciplinary action if it is considered fee splitting, a kickback, or a rebate to the PPMC. This action by the Florida Board of Medicine is being held in abeyance while being appealed and reviewed by the Florida District Court of Appeals, a procedure that will take approximately one year. To complicate the situation further, as reported in the April 22, 1998, issue of the *Wall Street Journal*, the Inspector General's Office of the U.S. Department of Health and Human Services raised similar concerns in an advisory opinion. Most people believe, however, that the investor model physician management company will either win the case outright, demonstrating that it is not in the "fee splitting" business, or will change the relationship with the physician's group to accommodate the law. The bottom line is that there is no real belief that the growth in PPMCs will be significantly curtailed as a consequence of this legal challenge.

Therefore, typically the MSO corporation provides management services to medical groups for a fee and serves as the contracting entity for managed care contracts. If the MSO is successful in controlling costs and in obtaining managed care contracts, it can generate a profit for itself and its investors. As a result of the potential for profits and stock appreciation, capital can be raised through outside investors. Physicians who enter into such a PPMC agreement must give up their practice assets, and, if they become unhappy with the group, they must begin anew without assets and are subject to noncompete covenants.

We seem to be moving away from autonomy in independent medical practices through the concept of practice sharing, IPAs, and group practices without walls and moving into the multispecialty group mode, with or without outside investors, and seeking to become a fully integrated delivery systems and major players in the marketplace.

In the broad array of often confounding practice opportunities that present themselves to physicians, there is a multiplicity of determinants that relate not only to the stage of managed care market evolution but also to issues of autonomy, compensation, quality of life, and the stage of practice life of the physician.

There are three distinctive phases in a physician's career. In the early phase are house staff members, right out of residency, who are usually looking for security, coverage, quality of life, and stability. At the opposite end of the spectrum are physicians who are five to 10 years away from retirement and who want to maximize their financial benefits and explore various take-out strategies. In the middle, of course, are people who have 20 or more years left in practice, the ones who struggle most with these complex options.

Each individual must evaluate the amount of financial risk he or she is willing to take and the amount of autonomy he or she needs versus financial stability and job security.

Physician Practice Acquisition and Alignment: Who Has the Advantage?

There are pluses and minuses in the not-for-profit hospital-physician relationship. The pluses are the potential alignment of cultural values and physician comfort in getting together with a hospital with which they have had a good relationship as a medical staff member. The minuses, as mentioned before, are that these relationships have not been very successful. Hospital management and board are in control, because physicians cannot control the board of trustees. Often, the hospital does not have the right set of management skills for doing physician practice management.

As for an alignment with or a sale to an investor-owned hospital, the plus side is that the stock market, at least for the present, creates the ability for ready capitalization, the tendency for purchase prices some 5-7 times earnings before income tax (EBIT), and the potential for managed care contracts. The minus primarily relates to a high probability of conflicting agendas between physicians and the hospital.

Finally, the plus side of an investor-owned physician practice management company (PPMC) is that it tends to be physician-oriented, and there is major physician participation in governance. In a friendly stock market, capitalization is relatively easy and has the potential for capturing managed care contracts on a regional, even national, level. The major minus at the moment is that there are very narrow financial margins in physician practice. Therefore, continuous growth is an absolute necessity in order to keep Wall Street happy.

Operating Margin on Physician Organizations

When physicians are a component of an integrated health care system, i.e., a hospital system, operating margins are generally negative—very negative in the Northwest, at 8 percent, and less negative in the Western systems, at about 2.3 percent. However, if you look at certain physician management companies, the margins, although relatively narrow, are still positive, for example, 6.5 percent for PhyCor.

Physician Practice Management Companies

As recently as late 1997, Salomon Brothers, a major New York-based investment firm, predicted that the growth of publicly traded PPMCs would reach an approximate $20 billion market in the ensuing five years. They felt that the key to success would be both market share expansion and, more important, demonstrable improvement in clinical practices that would promote lower delivery and operating costs. In other words, it would promote significant "same store" growth.

Rise of the Physician Practice Management Business Niche

The number of publicly traded PPMCs grew from only three in 1992 to 27 in 1996 and to 30 in 1998. In late 1996, total revenue for PPMCs had grown to more than $5 billion, with PhyCor leading this growth. As a consequence, there has been a great increase in the number of physicians whose practices are owned and managed by physician management companies.

How Does All This Look to Wall Street?

Until early 1998, the PPMC industry was one of the "darlings" of Wall Street. This is very significant, because Wall Street is the major source of equity financing for the growth of these companies. About 28 of the 30 PPMCs posted earning increases. Despite this, Wall Street remained concerned about the entire PPMC concept.

Wall Street's concerns were confirmed when, suddenly, the potential merger of two major PPMCs (PhyCor and MedPartners) collapsed. This was followed by the demise of a number of potential major deals between PPMCs and major clinics that had been in the works for years. Wall Street's response was evident when PPMC stocks fell from 40 to 90+ percent, which resulted in bankruptcy of some PPMCs and withdrawal of others, such as MedPartners, from the physician management business.

How this will evolve in the near future is anyone's guess. Currently, despite these major setbacks, there is a growing consensus that there is an important place for PPMCs and that they will search for a different way to do business. Those that are well managed will develop refocusing survival techniques. The industry leader, PhyCor, has changed some of its methodology and appears prepared to ride out these rough waters over the long term, because a functional physician organization in this highly competitive marketplace is a necessity.

Relative to this issue, Uwe Reinhardt, a Princeton University economics professor, has described what he calls the securitization of patients.[3] "Securitization of a thing is the formal sale of ownership rights in the future cash flow likely to be thrown off by that thing." Businesses are securitized through the sale of ownership certificates called "common stock." He goes on to state that, from a financial perspective, patients can be viewed as "biological structures that yield future net cash flows." Whoever can claim legal title to these net cash flows can securitize and resell them in the open market. For example, Reinhardt says, commercial managed care plans view an insured life as a future net cash yield equal to the annual premium per insured life minus the plan's outlays for the insured's medical care, or the so-called "medical loss ratio." For physicians in a medical practice rendering patient care under fee-for-service compensation, the net cash flow inherent in patient care is the gross revenue generated by whatever treatments the physician renders the patient minus the cost of providing those treatments. The PPMC's ability to securitize is key to Wall Street.

Practice Purchasing Valuation

Practices are valued on their earnings before income tax (EBIT), and a purchase offer is made somewhere around 4-6 times that figure. For example, if a practice's net collections are $800,000 and the estimated operating expenses before physician payments are $400,000 (again, about 50 percent of net collectibles are the cost of doing business), a net to the practice of $400,000 is left. If the physician's compensation is $340,000, that leaves an EBIT of $60,000. The PPMC would offer four to six times that, or $240,000 to $360,000, for the purchase of the practice, in addition to the hard assets of the practice, such as leases, equipment, etc. More recently, these multiples have significantly decreased as PPMCs have fallen on hard times.

In addition to these up-front payments, the physician agrees to work for the PPMC on a salaried basis with a contract that prohibits the selling physician from competing directly with the acquiring company should the employment contract be terminated. The PPMC, after purchasing several hundred of these practices, can resell the pooled cash flow on Wall Street for a multiple of six to eight times the EBIT. The acquiring company's shareholders profit from this arbitrage.

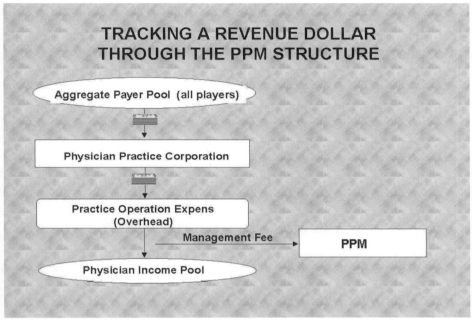

TRACKING A REVENUE DOLLAR THROUGH THE PPM STRUCTURE

Aggregate Payer Pool (all players)

Physician Practice Corporation

Practice Operation Expens (Overhead)

Management Fee → PPM

Physician Income Pool

Figure 10

Therefore, after the sale to the PPMC is consummated and the management company has purchased some or all of the tangible assets and has created a long-term management agreement for somewhere between 20 and 40 years, the following operational revenue scheme frequently pertains relative to the managed care contracts that the PPMC brings to the practices (figure 10, above). The money comes in at the top; the PPMC corporation takes its cut off the top for bringing in the money, and then the dollars flow to the cost of running the practices. An additional cost is then taken off by the PPMC local management company, which is offering MSO services to the physician practices (usually somewhere in the range of 10-15 percent), and the remainder goes into the physician income pool to support physician salaries and bonus arrangements. In addition, this physician income pool is often split between the physicians and the PPMC. Splits vary from group to group, with a range of 10-15 percent going to the PPMC. In this kind of scheme, physicians may have an ownership position in the PPMC and an ownership position in the MSO function and may receive income from the physician income pool. In general, PPMCs leave physicians in control of issues relative to the practice of medicine and focus their attention on managing tangible practice assets, such as receivables, contracts, information systems, medical equipment, and real estate leases.

As noted earlier, these traditional methodologies of physician practice purchase are now being modified significantly by:

- Reducing practice prices.

- Shortening the management agreement.

- Reducing capital expenditures on acquired practices.

- Expanding existing practices, working on "same store" efficiencies, and improving customer service.

The bottom line is that successful PPMCs must show that they can consistently run practices better and add value by bringing new business to those practices, especially from the managed care sector.

Rating the Advantages of PPMCs

There are both advantages and disadvantages of physicians' entering into such financial arrangements with PPMCs. The capital formation element is very positive, because physicians gain easy access to investment capital. Usually, PPMCs come with well-organized, state-of-the-art information systems and bring better business management than the physician practice previously had. In addition, there is a promise and a delivery on getting managed care contracts, from both regional and national carriers. If the venture is successful, the physician will profit through stock ownership. Physicians have a major voice in the control of medical decisions, especially on the local level, but they must meet corporate financial goals at the same time. Long-term control over the destiny of the group is minimal; in fact, the group could be totally sold as a package to another PPMC, or to Benson and Hedges. The new owners could have a totally different cultural and management style. This issue of one PPMC gobbling up another is far from hypothetical.

It is obvious, therefore, that physicians currently face many complicated decisions. However, if they decide to move more closely into the corporate practice of medicine through networking arrangements, employment arrangements, group practice arrangements, or aligning with or selling out to PPMCs, they cannot protest too vigorously that they ended up in a commercial model, that their employer sees patients as merely a revenue stream, or that they're being forced to make financial decisions rather than clinical decisions. By deciding to move along this integration continuum, physicians have consciously converted their practices into the commercial model, in return for large up-front payments, the potential of increasing personal wealth through the Wall Street venue, and establishing long-term job security. Dr. Reinhardt ends his article, "Hippocrates did not speak to these aspects of professional ethics because he did not even contemplate such deals."

Components of an Integrated Delivery System (IDS)

For all the reasons stated earlier relative to the national push stimulating mergers, consolidations, and alignments, the current thrust is toward creating a variety of highly complex, integrated delivery systems. It is entirely possible to have physician hospital organizations, MSOs networking with IPAs, mixed models, group and staff models of physicians involving academic teaching centers and hospitals, as well as alternative delivery sites or MSOs linking a variety of physician practice models. As a result, health systems are integrating horizontally (to create economies of scale, market leverage, and coverage of large geographic areas) and vertically (to offer economies of scope and cost-effectiveness across the system by bringing together all modes of health care service). Although the jury is still out on how effective these IDSs will be, the conventional wisdom that some forms of IDS have value and that the benefits are real and desirable is pushing providers into these types of integrated systems. Through this type of integration, improvements in cost-effectiveness can be achieved, disease management protocols can be implemented across the continuum of care, and appropriate market synergies can be developed. However, accomplishing these goals requires a lot of work by management and a major acculturation of the various participants.

It is reasonable to predict that, once integrated provider organizations have fully mastered the task of managing risk, they will be tempted to form what is now being called provider-sponsored organizations (PSOs) or provider-sponsored networks (PSNs). These organizations are capable of contracting directly with government, large private employers, or associations of small employers. The goal is to eliminate the insurance industry as the middleman between the payer and the provider and to capture for providers profits now being earned by the middleman. Not surprisingly, for precisely these reasons, the insurance industry is unlikely to be supportive of such PSO initiatives.

By definition, PSOs are integrated networks of physicians, hospitals, pharmacies, and other allied health care facilities capable of assuming full financial risk for the cost of a group of insured patients. PSOs deal with enrolled patient populations. They can go directly to self-insured employers or business coalitions and, as Medicare modifications continue, directly to Medicare beneficiaries. Recent Florida legislation has opened up Medicaid to PSOs, without requiring an HMO license. The provider is directly involved in defining the scope of benefit; this is a vehicle that puts the PSO, and therefore providers, at risk. The providers get to set the reimbursement schedule but, in order to succeed, they must manage utilization, cost infrastructure, stop-loss reinsurance, and out-of-area coverage. In the PSO format, provider, not the managed care organization, establish performance standards and must have very sophisticated information systems.

HCFA and PSOs: Certification Process

The certification process to create a PSO is a long and winding road through a very, very difficult bureaucratic process that could take up to a year and a half to complete. It is believed that, in an approved PSO, providers must control at least 51 percent of the equity; that a controlling interest may be held by only one provider; that the PSO will be required to demonstrate that at least 70 percent of its services are offered by its ownership providers; and that the PSO must demonstrate at least $1.5 million dollars in reserves to satisfy solvency requirements. How liquid this $1.5 million must be is currently being debated.

Equity and governance are shared between physicians and hospitals in a PSO, which contracts with managed care organizations, employers, and government to provide services to employees and subscribers. In order to achieve this, through a risk-contracting percentage of premium, the PSO would subcontract its services to a physician network made up of primary care physicians and specialists in various network configurations. It would also have contracts for services, discounted or capitated, with hospitals, alternative sites, diagnostic facilities, home care agencies, etc. Not surprisingly, they would have to have the same back-room functions as those currently housed in a managed care organization dealing with contracting—practice management, billing and claims, group purchasing, finance and accounting, marketing, information systems, planning, network development, utilization review/quality assurance, and total quality management, for example.

It is hoped that, as a result of PSOs, responsibility for effective clinical decision making will move from managed care plans and their distant "1-800-MAY-I" utilization management nurses to community physicians who are both local and at risk. As risk is accepted by these provider enterprises, so will be responsibility for setting appropriate clinical standards and mechanisms for policing these standards. Through PSOs, it is hoped that physicians will be able to develop stable organizational structures capable of restoring clinical autonomy to physicians. It is also hoped that physicians can again nurture the general public's trust in them and in these organizations.

In sum, the concept of providers creating their own organizations (PSOs) to contract directly with government for Medicare lives seems ideal, because they could not only regain control of the marketplace, make key decisions, and better manage care but also turn profits. PSOs could secure 100 percent of the Medicare premium dollar themselves, cutting out the MCO middleman and pocketing the 15-20 percent premium that MCOs took profit and administrative costs. So, in this PSO concept, one is talking about the potential of significant dollars, but also highly significant risk, as evidenced by the recent failure of two HCFA PSO demonstration projects.

There is a downside to all this, however. An incisive editorial in the *Annals of Internal Medicine* quoted Pogo and stated, "We have met the enemy and he is us!" It warned that if physicians in PSOs adopt, without modification, the same mechanisms and values currently utilized by managed care organizations to control prices and utilization, they will resemble these managed care organizations and will not have differentiated themselves from managed care organizations as had been hoped.[4]

The latter part of 1998 was not very positive for large, complex enterprises. Integrated delivery systems, such as Columbia/HCA, the Allegheny Health Education and Research Foundation, Kaiser Permanente, etc., have not thrived. In addition, there has been a failure to create a consistently workable strategy for organizing physicians. Acquisition of physician practices has generally been financially disastrous. Yet, solo practices and independent groups are also finding it difficult to maintain income, to raise capital, and to meet their infrastructure needs. As noted, the for-profit PPMC sector has imploded, with financial losses, litigation, and even bankruptcy.

In conclusion, I think it is fair to say that the complete professional autonomy that the individual American physician has traditionally enjoyed in health care is a thing of the past. Physicians will have to accommodate to the fact that, in their daily work, clinical decisions are going to be monitored and constrained by some organization, be it run by nonphysicians or, ideally, by a new generation of physician organizations. The key question is whether physicians, as a group, will be ruled by the insurance industry through managed care under a divide-and-conquer principle, as is the case today, or whether, by organizing themselves, they can topple the insurance industry from its current position of power and make it subservient to the dictates of provider-managed PSOs. There is hope that organized medicine and physicians individually can rise to this challenge; reverse the power curve back to the supply side; and, thereby, return professionalism to the doctor/patient relationship.

However, there must be significant concern when we mix money, medicine, and ethics. The doctor/patient relationship must be shielded from the influence of these raw market forces. The relationship between the patient and the physician is one of service, vulnerability, and collaboration and must be protected from conflicting financial interests that may jeopardize the vulnerable patient. Commercial interests can bias even the most devoted professional, and care must be taken to guard against such bias. Physician alignments raise ethical concerns regarding the effect of a shared economic interest among hospitals. To whom do financial arrangements ally a physician—the people being served, or the people paying for health care?

The current emphasis in the health care industry on structure, economic incentives, physician alignments, and general management does, in some cases, divert attention from the critical decision-making role of the physician acting on the behalf of his or her patient. We know that market forces may create economic efficiencies, but they do not guarantee sound, ethical values and, in fact, frequently act to the contrary. This issue must be kept foremost in physicians' minds. They must protect themselves from temptations that could bias them more toward financial reward than toward being patient advocates.

References

1. Weiner, J. "Forecasting the Effects of Health Reform on U.S. Physician Workforce Requirement. Evidence from HMO Staffing Patterns." *JAMA* 272(3):222-30, July 1994.

2. Japsen, B. "The Reluctant Doctors." *Modern Healthcare* 27(35):66,68, Sept. 1, 1997.

3. Reinhardt, U. "Economics: Hippocrates and the 'Securitization' of Patients." *JAMA* 277(23):1850-1, June 18, 1997.

4. Griner, P. "Residency Overwork and Changing Paradigms of Service." *Annals of Internal Medicine* 123(7):54, Oct. 1, 1995.

CHAPTER 4

Work Force Issues

Situation Wanted
Well-Trained Physician Seeks Professional Opportunity

Not a typical ad today, but it's generally believed that the United States is on the verge of a serious oversupply of physicians. In the March 6, 1996, edition of *JAMA*, there was, for the first time, some real data, not just anecdotal, that some physicians attempting to enter practices, in some specialties, in some regions of the country, are beginning to experience difficulty. In some cases, up to 10 percent of resident physicians were unable to find full-time positions in their specialties or subspecialties. This was especially evident in anesthesiology, gastroenterology, radiology, cardiovascular disease, and plastic surgery.[1] Because of these results, the study was repeated in 1996, with results published in the June 4, 1997, *JAMA*. The bottom line was essentially the same: "Results regarding the 1995 graduates are consistent with those obtained regarding the 1994 graduates and continue to suggest that the market for physician services, in some disciplines, continues to be restrictive."[2]

This seems to be a dynamic situation. The specialties of anesthesiology and plastic surgery, which had great difficulty in finding acceptable positions in 1994, had less difficulty in 1995. In 1995, the fields in which physicians had the greatest difficulty in finding employment included nephrology, pulmonary disease, critical care medicine, and endocrinology. A number of people believe that there will be progressive increases in the percentage of graduates who experience difficulties in finding suitable professional opportunities in their specialties or subspecialties.

Having had the opportunity and pleasure of relating with medical students for a number of years, I have noted that, early on in medical school, a significant portion of every class begins to struggle with the problem of what field of medicine to pursue. This sometimes occurs as early as the first year. With each year, the percentage of students pondering this issue grows in a logarithmic manner so that, by the end of the second year, prior to beginning clinical clerkships, the subject of which field of medicine to pursue becomes a frequent subject of discussion among medical students and their professors.

The reality is that all new physicians have to make a definitive decision on which broad field to become involved with. This is not a theoretical or academic exercise, but rather a major career lock-in, because the decision occurs with the National Intern and Resident Matching Plan (NIRMP) for the PGY I year, which always seems to happen sooner than one might expect. Parenthetically, despite the recently noted "bugs" in the algorithm used by NIRMP, the program works quite well overall and appears to be slightly biased toward the selection of the student.

This career decision has always been difficult for students because of inadequate data as to the nature of the various disciplines and because students are not really sure of their true interests or skills. Not infrequently, the decision is made by process of elimination.

Finally, slightly more than 50 percent of new physicians look for practice opportunities in the geographic area in which they train. However, a high percentage of the geographically more desirable practice locations are oversaturated. Therefore, despite the fact that more than 50 percent of residents try to find a practice opportunity in the area in which they have received their graduate medical education training, more and more residency programs are injecting "restrictive covenants" as part of acceptance into the residency training program. A "restrictive covenant" essentially states that once you have finished your residency, you agree not to practice within a specified geographic area, sometimes within a 50-mile radius, other times within a set of counties. When scouting potential residency programs, the new physician should inquire about such "restrictive covenants."

Compounding the problem are broad issues of lifestyle and family life, as well as compensation expectations. One should not be embarrassed or ashamed about the fact that the expectation of a relatively secure financial future has been an element of attraction for many top college students to enter the medical profession. In the past, it was true that cognitive or primary care physicians earned less than procedure-based specialty groups, and it has been suggested by some that such potential earning capacity influenced specialty choice. However, we all are aware that, with the continuing changes in the health care system, both the relative and the absolute earnings of medical generalists and specialists will be significantly affected. A concrete and meaningful example of income shifts results from the Balanced Budget Act of 1997, wherein Medicare moved to a single conversion factor. This simple shift, in effect, redistributes millions of dollars among physicians, so that there are major decreases in surgical specialties and modest increases in primary care specialties, such as internal medicine and family practice.

Physician Income

There was a progressive increase in the median income of physicians until 1994, when the first decrease, from $156,000 to $150,000, was noted. However, the figure rebounded in 1995 to $160,000 (figure 1, page 67).

The most recent compensation report shows that physician compensation is continuing to rise, despite the forces of managed care and concerns about an oversupply of doctors. However, only nine of 14 specialties enjoyed gains.[3]

It is now believed that the penetration of managed care and the regional supply of

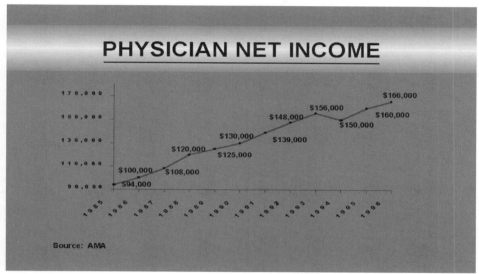

Figure 1

physicians does, indeed, follow the normal market forces of supply and demand. That is, the payers of health care are able to ratchet down payments to providers (physicians and hospitals) when there is a perceived excess capacity of these providers in a geographic area (figure 2, below).

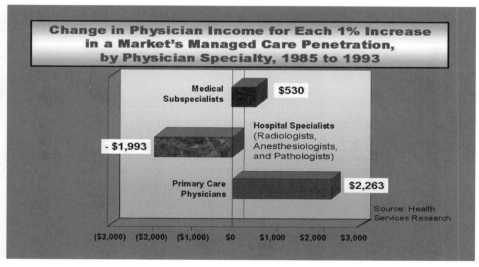

Figure 2

There is a very high ratio of physicians per 100,000 population in the same areas of the country in which there is high managed care penetration: California, Minnesota, New England, New York, and Florida. These areas have between 25 percent and 45 percent market penetration of managed care. On the contrary, managed care penetration is less than 3 percent in South Dakota and Alaska, and these states have some of the lowest ratios of physicians per 100,000 population.

Physician Income Is Related to Managed Care

Median physician incomes lessen in higher managed care areas. A number of studies have concluded that there is an inverse correlation between physician income and the amount of managed care penetration in any given geographic area.

What this means and how to interpret it are as iffy as predicting the weather for next week. However, most observers believe that increased managed care translates into decreased physician payments, which is compounded by increased costs of running a medical practice; physicians' net incomes across the board will go down, and specialists will experience the impact more than generalists.

In addition, over the past decade, there has been a marked decrease in the number of physicians in solo practice and a significant increase in the number of employed physicians—to approximately 40 percent of the total. The most recent data, from 1995, show that some 45.4 percent, or almost half, of all practicing physicians are now in some employment relationship. These new data stimulated the head of the American Medical Association to comment, "Anyone going into medicine today needs to understand that it is a rapidly changing environment, and you may not be your own boss."[4] It is being postulated that managed care, along with the growing physician supply, are the major forces stimulating new doctors to become employees in larger group practices, rather than facing the risk of starting smaller, private, solo practices.

Medicine is moving away from unit pricing, the so-called fee-for-service approach, to marketplace capitation and away from a more autonomous, entrepreneurial "mom and pop" type provider network to a coalescing of large integrated delivery systems exemplified by Columbia, Tenet, CIGNA, Prudential, PhyCor, and other major national integrated delivery systems. These evolving systems and the move away from the old paradigm significantly affect the demand and compensation side of the work force equation.

Work Force Forecasting

The history in the United States of predicting health manpower and supply has proven to be imprecise and, in fact, inadequate. President Harry Truman, after WW II, initiated the first subsidization of health care by linking the GI Bill of Rights for thousands of returning U.S. servicemen to it, thereby making it possible for them to go to medical school through scholarships and loans.

Physician Supply

In 1953, after WW II, the president's commission on the health needs of the nation predicted a physician shortage, which was reaffirmed by the Bane Commission in 1959. As a consequence, two things happened:

- Congress opened the gates for international medical graduates to be admitted to the United States.

- Of equal significance, the number of positions for U.S. students almost doubled, increasing the number of medical schools as well as class sizes in existing schools through a variety of funding mechanisms.

By 1980, with the report of the Graduate Medical Education National Advisory Committee (GMENAC), the futurists reversed their predictions, stating there would be a physician glut, or an oversupply of some 70,000, by the year 1990 and an excess of approximately 145,000 by the year 2000. Subsequent studies, with the exception of the AMA study in 1988, have also concluded that there will be a physician glut (figure 3, below).

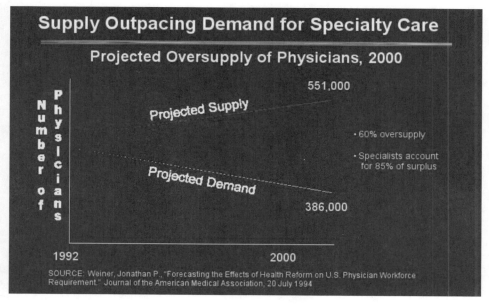

Figure 3

In 1995-1996, five additional and somewhat contradictory studies relative to health care work force were published. The most prominent perhaps is the report of the Pew Health Professionals Commission, which predicted an oversupply of physicians of some 100,000 to 150,000 out of the total of 600,000 they predicted would be practicing by the year 2000. The commission recommended the United States:

- Close enough medical schools to cut at least 20 percent of the first-year slots over the next decade.

- Limit residency slots to 110 percent of U.S. graduates.

- Tighten emigration restrictions on IMGs.

- Steer at least 50 percent of physicians into primary care residencies by the year 2000.

- Provide at least 25 percent of clinical training in ambulatory, community, and managed care sites.

- Create an all-payer pool to fund medical education.

A Council on Graduate Medical Education's (COGME) report, in 1995, stated that there was an excess of physicians but only in certain specialties. The report indicated there was a supply and demand balance for primary care physicians. The major problem was related to residency programs, where there was a significant excess of international medical graduates.

The Institute of Medicine reported, through a committee on the U.S. physician supply, that the large and rising numbers of physicians in this nation will face negative consequences unless some concrete steps are taken soon. The recommendations were:

- No new schools of allopathic or osteopathic medicine.

- Decreased federal funding for graduate medical education, bringing support for first-year residency slots close to the current number of U.S. medical graduates.

- Government steps to find replacement funding for IMG-dependent hospitals.

- Cooperation between the AMA and other professional associations and the federal government to widely disseminate information on physician supply and career opportunities in medicine to medical students and other interested parties.

The SACHS Group reported, in 1996, that there was a specialist surplus; however, at that same time, it reported a marked generalist shortage.

Finally, in the November 1996 issue of *JAMA*, the need to project wide geographic variations was noted, along with the need to emphasize benchmarking when analyzing physician supply and imbalance.

To add more confusion to the debate, COGME, in 1997, made some new recommendations:

- Cap medical education funding for residents at the 1996 residency numbers.

- Unlink payment to hospitals for indirect medical education from the number of residents.

- Phase down funds for international medical graduates over a number of years to zero, phase out the J1 Visas, and require those with J1 Visas to return to their countries of origin in five years after arriving in the United States.

- Provide medical education funding for ambulatory care sites.

In addition, a coalition of national medical and academic organizations issued a consensus statement at the end of February 1997. The group was made up of AMA, AAMC, American Association of the College of Osteopathic Medicine, American Osteopathic Association, Association of Academic Health Centers, and National Medical Association. The group's recommendations were to keep residency positions closely aligned with the number of graduates of accredited U.S. medical schools and to do this by limiting federal funding of graduate medical education to that number, focusing again on international medical graduate issues. It is expected that the National Bipartisan Commission on the Future of Medicare will also make major work force recommendations.

In spite of the confusing and variable data they have presented, there have been many work force forecasting models developed over time. There have been supply-side models, needs-based models, demand-based models, and econometric models. All of them, in one way or another, are seriously flawed, because many of the assumptions utilized to create the models are inaccurate. Moreover, there is a serious lack of data needed to drive the models.

Forecasting of work force numbers will always be very imprecise at best. Therefore, be very skeptical about predictions of the future relative to numbers and types of physicians necessary, and do not link the future of your professional lives on soft and ever-changing data. However, forecasting is not as important as the impact of the market itself on the demand for specific types of health care workers in specific local markets.

Market Forces

The major current market force is managed care and it keeps growing, now enrolling in excess of 80 million people, approximately one quarter of the U.S. population. Although this growth has not been equally distributed among all the states, just about every state has had some activity. Like hospitals in managed care-intense markets, which are experiencing decreasing occupancy and significantly decreasing lengths of stay, specialists are on the endangered species list where managed care has been growing; only a small percentage of existing specialists in these markets is needed to serve managed care enrollees.

Growth in Filled Residency Training Programs

There has been a significant and progressive increase in the total number of physicians in residency training in the United States, growing from approximately 85,000 to approximately 105,000 in the past six years. It is obvious that these residency training positions are the pipeline to place physicians into the marketplace.

From 1979 to 1996, there was a progressive increase in the total number of allopathic residents, from approximately 65,000 to about 100,000 residents (figure 4, below).

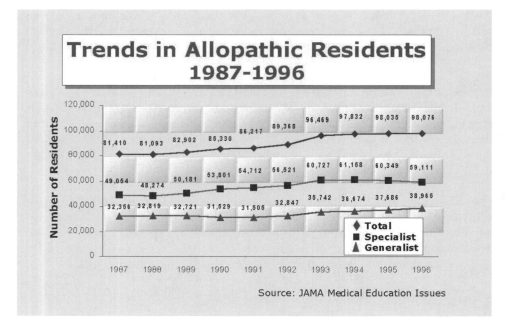

Source: JAMA Medical Education Issues

Figure 4

There has been significant growth in the absolute number of physicians, as well as in the number of physicians per 100,000 population. In the 1950s and 1960s, there were slightly more than 600,000 physicians in the United States, or approximately 140 physicians per 100,000 population. This has grown to close to 800,000 physicians in the United States, or approximately 240 physicians per 100,000 population. It is projected that, if no major new policies are enacted, there will be approximately 900,000 physicians in the United States by the year 2020, which equates to 275 physicians per 100,000 population.

Current FTE staffing estimates of physicians in HMOs range from 112 physicians per 100,000 population to a high of 138 physicians per 100,000 population. The fee-for-service sector shows a need for 207 physicians per 100,000 population. Whether they view the issue from the fee-for-service model or more starkly from the perspective of managed care, most experts now agree that the aggregate physician supply is moving toward a significant overload. Whether an overload of physicians is "good" or "bad" depends on one's economic philosophy. In addition to physician supply, one cannot overlook other elements that add to significant imbalances. There is now general agreement that there are too many specialists compared to generalists, that there are too few physicians in rural areas and in inner cities, and that there is an under-representation of minorities in the physician work force. Other complicating factors have to be added to the equation, such as increasing the number of nonphysician providers—i.e., nurse practitioners and physician assistants—as well as the issue of international medical graduates.

Despite the uncertainty and inexact science of forecasting work force requirements, the following are believed to be truisms:

- U.S. medical schools graduate more than 16,000 people per year.

- Over time, the number of applicants for those medical school positions gradually rose, from almost 43,000 applicants in 1993 to approximately 47,000 applicants in 1994. In 1997, the applicant pool fell to 43,000 students. It was estimated that, in 1998, the figure would fall to 41,000, approximately a 12.5 percent decline from the peak year. Nonetheless, these applicants are still significantly more than the 16,000 positions available. Most people in academic medicine believe that, at the 47,000 level, the applicant field was probably too high, and we are now reaching the right balance.

- To compound the work force problem, there is a continued influx of international medical graduates to the United States, at least in part stimulated by the service requirements of inner-city teaching hospitals. In 1995, 23.5 percent of all practicing physicians were IMGs.

- In managed care systems, there is increasing utilization of nonphysician providers and continuously expanding roles for these providers. These individuals are not only nurse practitioners and physician assistants but also psychologists, pharmacists, optometrists, and others. For example, in the Twin Cities in Minnesota, an area in which managed care is highly evolved, HealthPartners (a system caring for some 700,000 members) comprises 350 employed physicians, of which 250 are primary care physicians, utilizing some 20 medical sites. In addition to primary care physicians, this group uses adult nurse practitioners, pediatric nurse practitioners, physician assistants, OB/GYN nurse practitioners, and nurse midwives. The trend is toward increasing the role of nursing both at the mid-level and at the nurse practitioner level. HealthPartners created health care teams made up of physicians, nurses, nurse practitioners, physician assistants, psychologists, and clinical pharmacists, which translates to 50 physicians per 100,000 population. With this example in mind, it is easy to understand that increased managed care will result in a real change in the work force configurations that will deliver it in the future.

- There is a growing commitment nationally to embrace the concept of the so-called "50-percent solution." That is, the percentage of medical graduates entering the primary care disciplines of family medicine, general internal medicine, and general pediatrics should increase from the current levels of 25-30 percent to at least 50 percent by the year 2000. Several states have already enacted laws requiring their medical schools to graduate half of their classes in primary care disciplines. Many of the health reform proposals before Congress had similar language. Although these legislative pieces did not pass, the conventional wisdom of the 50-percent solution has persisted.

The 50/50 approach is not based on a lot of hard data; it is an expression of social policy, a call for work force balance. As a consequence of this social pressure and political policy, for the seventh year in a row, more graduating U.S. medical students have chosen primary care for their first-year residency positions. In the 1999 match of U.S. medical school seniors, 54 percent chose generalist specialties: family practice, internal medicine, and pediatrics. The remaining 46 percent chose surgical specialties, psychiatry, OB/GYN, etc. However, it is important to note that the 1996 AAMC Medical School Graduation Questionnaire revealed that only approximately 30 percent of the graduating students intended to pursue careers as primary care physicians.

A landmark piece of research done by Jonathan Weiner of John's Hopkins School of Public Health, Baltimore, Maryland, is accepted as a benchmark for work force policy projections.[5] The basic assumption of the study was that 40-60 percent of Americans would receive care from managed care programs in the near future and that most Americans would be covered by some type of health insurance. Weiner then developed three alternative scenarios:

- Twenty percent of U.S. medical graduates would enter primary care.

- The proportion would increase to the 50/50 solution.

- The current number of residency positions would be scaled back to 110 percent of the number of U.S. graduates.

From these assumptions, Weiner came to the following conclusions:

- The overall supply of physicians will significantly outstrip requirements, with a surplus estimated to equal 50 physicians per 100,000 population, or 165,000 excess physicians.

- The primary care physician supply would be in equilibrium. (This conclusion was reconfirmed by Whitcomb.[6])

- Under all scenarios, there would be a significant surplus of specialists, ranging between 60 and 75 percent above requirements by the year 2000. A recent COGME report estimated the excess to be about 100 specialists per 100,000 population, or some 125,000 specialists.

Faced with these issues, the United States must make a choice. It can look to the market to recalibrate its work force, or it can attempt to manage it more directly. This debate and dilemma will continue for the next few years. There will be two schools of thought. One will advocate, "Don't dictate to medical students; let the market take care of the need for practitioners." Another school will advocate, "Given that the federal government is the major underwriter of graduate medical education, it would only seem prudent that active management of total physician supply become a national priority."

Under the first scenario, the marketplace theories are as follows:

- If there are not enough doctors in rural America, educate more physicians, and maybe more of them will trickle out to rural areas.

- If there are not enough doctors practicing in the inner city, educate more physicians, and maybe the oversupply in the metropolitan market will force more to practice in the inner city.

- If not enough doctors choose to go into primary care, maintain the size of medical school enrollment and saturate the technological specialties, and maybe more physicians will enter primary care specialties.

It follows that, if traditionally more glamorous and more highly paid specialties are overcrowded, the marketplace will squeeze doctors into rural, inner-city, and primary care practices. These physicians will move to where they are needed and where demand still exists for their services. The rationale for supporting market forces is that any decision to artificially limit access to a particular occupation is antithetical to democratic free choice of careers in the United States.

Despite all of the theories and debates, the following findings seem to be true:

- The supply of physicians has continued to increase much faster than the U.S. population for the past 20 years.

- Market forces, enhanced by the growth of managed care, seem to have decreased the aggregate number of physicians required to deliver such services.

- Despite an abundance of physicians, many Americans do not have adequate access to health care. Access is a real problem for the 40+ million Americans who have no or inadequate health insurance coverage;

- The supply and demand theory hasn't worked, because there continues to be a shortage of generalists in inner-city areas and rural communities, despite the excess of physicians in general.

- The profusion of physicians in some specialties and subspecialties has not prompted an influx of physicians into primary care fields.

- Managed care plans, especially in areas in which capitation is more prominent, typically require fewer physicians than traditional indemnity plans, and discounted fee-for-service payment has forced physicians to increase patient volume in order to maintain their income, further reducing the total number of physicians required overall. This continued pressure to maximize productivity and reduce costs may mean less time for physicians to spend with each patient, which increases the potential for shoddy service and misdiagnoses, as well as diminished career satisfaction among physicians.

Moreover, the free market solution to manpower distribution has an additional major problem: about 250,000 American physicians might well be trained with skills that they might not be able to utilize appropriately after spending years attaining those skills and incurring significant debt. As a consequence, there is a need for a national health work force policy that combines legislative, regulatory, and voluntary incentives:

- Keep the number of PGY physicians pegged to approximately 110 percent of U.S. graduates. This, of course, has some flaws, because a large number of IMGs are U.S. citizens. Therefore, it would be difficult to deny them re-entry into this country.

- Close 20-25 percent of U.S. medical schools, and reduce the number of entering students by an equivalent amount by the year 2005. To effect such a move would be very difficult politically. It is doubtful that medical schools, especially publicly supported medical schools, are going to decrease their enrollment, especially as there continues to be a high demand for medical school admission by highly qualified undergraduates.

- Increase the number of residents in primary care by at least 50 percent. Although this is an attractive concept, and there has already been a significant shift of first-year slots toward primary care, one must be very cautious of moving too many physicians into primary care. There is growing evidence that patients with chronic diseases, such as cancer, diabetes, coronary artery disease, etc., will receive better care at a lower total cost if they are under the supervision of a specialist rather than a primary care physician.

None of these frequently suggested "cures" for the work force problem are totally workable solutions. Medicare Part A is the major mechanism for funding graduate medical education, and there have been some recent and serious debates on how it might be modified. Some significant provisions in the Balanced Budget Act of 1997 addressed Medicare funding of GME:

- It limits the number of total residencies for which Medicare will make payments.

- It will provide incentives for facilities to voluntarily reduce the number of residents they train.

New York state currently trains some 15 percent of the nation's housestaff, a large proportion of which are IMGs. In 1997, New York state academic centers, with the help of Senators Moynahan and D'Amato, were able to come to an agreement with HCFA to reduce the state's residencies by about 2,000 over six years while continuing to be compensated as if the residencies weren't cut. As a consequence, academic centers around the country wanted the same opportunity, and a provision to that effect was added to the Balanced Budget Act. Since that time, however, some 17 prominent New York hospitals have withdrawn from the voluntary program to reduce housestaff, and there is no indication that any other academic centers have opted to participate. It is important when looking at residency positions, therefore, to check out the status of the program to which you are applying.

As noted in the Balanced Budget Amendment of 1997, a National Bipartisan Commission on the Future of Medicare was created. It has met on a number of issues but is focusing on some issues that affect medical education, especially graduate medical education (GME). Some of the major focuses have been on "carving" direct GME payments and disproportionate share (DSH) hospital support out of Medicare and greatly reducing indirect medical education payments. The attempt here is to move these fiscal issues from Medicare to other elements of the federal budget so that they are still subject to annual appropriation debate. This approach raises great concerns, because there is no security in any annual appropriation process. The move is being vigorously opposed by the academic community.

The academic community, with support from some senators, is pursuing the establishment of a mandatory trust fund to support graduate medical education to which Medicare would continue to contribute. Other insurers would be required to be involved in supporting this newly formed trust fund. In addition, the Medicare Payment Advisory Commission (MedPAC) is involved in the debate about future funding of graduate medical education under Medicare and has focused significantly on the IMG issue. MedPAC noted that, in 1995, approximately 23.5 percent of all practicing physicians were IMGs, that some 70-75 percent of IMGs trained in the United States remain here after completing residencies, and that IMGs are disproportionately located in large cities with high non-Caucasian areas characterized by poverty and high infant mortality. Therefore, IMGs appear to be playing an important role as "safety nets."

To compound the issue, the vast majority of graduate medical education dollars go directly to teaching hospitals. There is a growing group of medical educators who believe that graduate as well as undergraduate medical education should be shifted from its inpatient/hospital focus to a more ambulatory focus, thereby reflecting current practice venues. There is a growing consensus that, if resident and student education are shifted to ambulatory sites, federal funds would also have to be shifted. This means hospitals would no longer control the funds, a concept the American Hospital Association would strongly oppose. So, there is growing support for the development of an "authorization system," such as funding vouchers for residents to provide payments to the site where the training is taking place.

The Balanced Budget Amendments

Now let's take a look at what happened in 1997 as a result of the Balanced Budget Amendments as the federal government begins to tinker with graduate medical education:

- Congress imposed a cap on the number of residents it will support through its direct and indirect teaching payments.

- Congress implemented a shift of medical education payments from managed care to teaching hospitals.

- The law extended GME payments for direct costs incurred by select ambulatory providers, such as federally qualified health centers, rural health clinics, and managed care plans that contract with Medicare.

- As mentioned earlier, the law also gave teaching hospitals the option to participate in residency downsizing programs similar to the one in New York.

Influential Republican political leaders have posed the following question concerning federal involvement in and tinkering with graduate medical education: Why should Medicare or other payers of health care services financially support institutions that train physicians? Similar organizations don't support graduate students in law, engineering, or business. Some believe we should establish a targeted voucher system or loan forgiveness program to support students who cannot afford to finance their medical education. This would place the government subsidy with individuals, where it belongs, rather than with institutions. This debate will continue to evolve. Its direction and the political climate in which it is conducted are still, of course, ill defined. Stay tuned.

Is it really so bad that physicians are polishing their CVs and resumes and preparing to enter into new lines of work? In a word, no. Why?

- Experts have been wrong in the past.

- The market adjusts. In other words, medical students, in selecting their graduate programs, have already begun to shift away from some programs that are believed to be over capacity into programs that are believed to be in more demand, such as primary care. In addition, a number of prestigious institutions have voluntarily decreased the number of their residency slots.

- Technology is the "X" factor. If the past is any predictor of the future, as new breakthroughs come online, more specialists will be needed to administer them.

- Pathologies never sleep. AIDS is only one of a series of emerging health care problems that are going to require a gamut of treatment specialists. Who knows what kinds of health problems, new viruses, or environmental hazards will emerge in the future?

- By the year 2030, the number of Americans age 65 years or older will double from 35 million to more than 70 million. This is the segment of the population that requires the greatest number of medical and surgical interventions.

- The consumer has not spoken. Although managed care is growing rapidly, one should not assume that the primary care gatekeeper model will prevail. It is also not safe to assume that patients will not demand more ready access to specialists when they believe they are necessary.

- Physicians, in 1996, were still in great demand in a number of very significant and attractive markets.

In the future, successful physicians will act more like managers. They will have to modify their culture and their behavior, especially moving from "what feels good" behavior to "more effective" behavior, from being a doer to becoming more of a planner, from one-to-one interactions to many interactions. This means being concerned with populations of patients rather than solely with individual patients. It means moving from immediate gratification to more delayed gratification, from being independent deciders to being delegaters, from pure autonomy to more collaboration. It means moving from independence to more participatory behavior.

It is also believed that more and more physicians will end up in organizational settings, such as in integrated delivery systems, and in the employ of organizations. More physicians will become salaried, and, as noted, more physicians will end up as physician executives/managers. Parenthetically, this is an area of significant growth, with an average compensation about 15-20 percent higher than average physician income.

Physicians must accept the major cultural change and move into a more effective behavior mode that will allow them to become organized and to assume an appropriate leadership role in reconfiguring the health care marketplace of the future. Because of that need for culture change and skills beyond those related to excellence in patient care, more and more academic programs are offering medical students and residents an opportunity to learn business skills so that they will be better prepared to practice in the evolving health care environment.

References

1. Miller, R.S. "The Initial Employment Status of Physicians Completing Training in 1994." *JAMA* 275(9):708-12, March 6, 1996.

2. Miller, R.S. "Initial Employment Status of Resident Physicians Completing Training in 1995." *JAMA* 277(21):1699-704, June 4, 1997 *JAMA*

3. *Physician Socioeconomic Statistics 1997.* Chicago, Ill.: American Medical Association, 1997.

4. James W. Todd, MD, Executive Vice President, American Medical Association, Chicago, Ill., personal communication, January 1997.

5. Weiner, J. "Forecasting the Effects of Health Reform on U.S. Physician Workforce Requirement. Evidence from HMO Staffing Patterns." *JAMA* 272(3):222-30, July 1994.

6. Whitcomb, M. "A Cross-National Comparison of Generalist Physician Workforce Data. Evidence for U.S. Supply Adequacy." *JAMA*. 274(9):692-5, Sept. 6, 1995.

CHAPTER 5

Physician Leadership for High Quality in a Price-Competitive World

by W. Michael Alberts, MD, MBA

Traditionally, quality has been hard to define. Some have even maintained that it cannot be defined. A formal definition from the Institute of Medicine is "the degree to which the process of care increases the probability of outcomes desired by patients and reduces the probability of undesired outcomes, given the state of medical knowledge."[1] A functional definition might be "health care that assists healthy people to stay healthy, cures people's acute illnesses, and allows chronically ill people to live as long and fulfilling lives as possible."

The Veteran's Administration defines high-quality health care as, "Care that is needed and delivered in a manner that is competent, caring, cost-effective, and timely and which minimizes risk and achieves achievable benefits."[2] "Needed" implies that the care was appropriate for that patient at that time. "Competent" means that care was delivered according to accepted standards. "Caring" means that the patient judged the care to be satisfactory. "Cost-effective" means that cost was factored into the decision-making process. "Timely" means that the care was given at the right time to accomplish the desired outcome or to meet patient expectations. "Minimizes risk" means that efforts were taken to protect the patient from harm. "Achieves achievable outcomes" means that an achievable positive outcome was the result of the care process.[2]

On a more philosophical note, however, quality is defined by the customer. Quality is "in the eye of the beholder." High quality, to a patient, means access and timeliness. High quality, to a physician, means achieving desirable outcomes. High quality, to a hospital, means financial viability and satisfied customers. High quality, to a payer, means lower costs and customer satisfaction. "High quality in a product or service is not what the provider puts in. It is what the consumer gets out and is willing to pay for. Consumers pay only for what is of use to them and gives them value. Nothing else is quality."[3]

There are two main dimensions of quality in health care: quality of service and quality of care. Quality of service means patient satisfaction. Quality of service may be termed "meeting and exceeding customer (patient) expectations." When the encounter meets patient expectations, the patient achieves a "quality in perception."[4] Patients' views of quality are shaped by their perception of three factors: institutional quality (corporate image in the public eye), physical quality (nice waiting room), and interactive quality (social interaction between staff, physician, and patient). There is no way to recover from lack of caring, rudeness, lack of enthusiasm, or other cues that signal poor quality to the patient. Quality of service is extremely important, because patients are often blind to quality of care. In general, they don't know if they've been given the correct antibiotic, or if they really needed a bronchoscopy. They use quality of service as a "surrogate" for quality of care. As a result, providers must put a great deal of emphasis on quality of service.

Quality of care is tremendously hard to define. It is sometimes termed "conformance to professional standards or technical specifications."[5] With such a definition, questions arise: Whose standards? Who judges conformance? Quality of care is thought to have two dimensions: appropriateness of the services provided and the skill with which the appropriate care is performed ("Doing the right thing right").[6] While acknowledging the difficulty in definition, most would agree that significant efforts to maximize and improve quality of care are warranted.

Assessment of Quality

As hard as it is to define, quality is even more difficult to measure. Yet, some sort of assessment is necessary in order to be able to manage it. You can manage only what you can measure.

Quality of Service

Quality of service is assessed by asking the customer (patient), "How am I doing?" Do we meet your access, availability, and convenience needs and preferences? In general, are we meeting your expectations? This information is usually acquired via patient satisfaction surveys. Although the patient is the obvious customer, do not forget other potential customers. Referring physician satisfaction, payer satisfaction, and staff satisfaction are important to the success of a practice. It is difficult to deliver excellent service if physicians, nurses, and other staff are unhappy. If a payer or a referring physician is unhappy, you won't need physicians, nurses, and other staff.

In addition to surveying the customer, it is also beneficial to measure quality of service indicators, such as time spent in the waiting room, availability of next appointment, and response time for telephone calls. Monitoring, assessing, and responding to patient complaints are key features of any quality management program. Remember that every complaint is a treasure. Most patients do not complain. They just do not return, and they tell all their friends, who tell all their friends. If patients don't complain, you never know you did not meet their expectations. As a result, you will miss an opportunity to prevent a similar circumstance from happening again.

Referring to the patient as a customer is offensive to some physicians. To me, this is mere semantics. In many ways, we actually honor patients by calling them customers. This places the patient as the focus of the relationship, rather than continuing the paternalistic interaction of the past, when the doctor was always right.

Like it or not, physicians of today are in the retail business. There are only two rules in retail: "the customer is always right," and "if the customer is wrong, refer to Rule 1."

Quality of Care

Quality of care is traditionally assessed by looking at structure, process, and outcome.[7] Structure is the resources assembled to deliver care. Process is "the care itself." Outcomes are the valued results of care.[8]

Structure is the work capacity of physicians, hospitals, and other components of the health care system. These are the essential features that must be present to deliver high-quality care. Their mere presence, however, does not ensure high quality. The analogy is that: you can try to analyze the performance of a car by using a checklist to verify the presence of an engine, brakes, headlights, etc. These features must be present, but their presence does not guarantee that the car will run. In health care, we might look at staffing ratios (physician to enrollee ratios), credentials (board certification), and accreditation (JCAHO, NCQA). Structure assessment attempts to answer the question: Do the providers have the knowledge, skills, and resources to diagnose and treat patients?

Process measures look at the interaction between a patient and his or her physician and at the treatment given, i.e., the series of events that occur in the provision of care. For example, one might look at rates of mammography, pap smears, and childhood immunizations. Additionally, one might use clinical practice guidelines to establish indicators to measure. For example, are smokers counseled on cessation? Are diabetics referred for ophthalmologic screening? Process measures are usually assessed via chart reviews and peer reviews.

An outcome describes the result of the care given on the individual's health. Examples might be sentinel events or sentinel diagnoses. Adverse outcomes, such as death during an elective surgery or admission for diabetic ketoacidosis, are flagged for further review. Clinical end points, such as mortality rate, readmission rate, or five-year survival rate, may serve as outcome measures.

Various measures of quality of life assessment may serve as outcomes measures. Functional status is a desired outcome and may, therefore, serve as a quality of life monitor. There are several types of functional status measurement, including physical, mental, social, and role function. Patient satisfaction is a crucial outcome. Aspects of satisfaction, such as access to care, convenience of delivery, and financial consideration, may be measured.

In fact, any aspect of quality may be examined with this structure, process, and outcome model. An example of structure measurement in asthma might be: Is spirometry available in the primary care practitioner's office? An example of process measure might be: Are inhaled steroids used in patients with more than mild asthma? An outcome measure might be the hospital admission rates for asthmatics.

Value = Quality/Cost

Value = Quality/Cost is a key concept. Purchasers of health care want to maximize value just as do purchasers of other items; we all want the most for our money. If one item costs more than another and the quality is the same, why not choose the cheaper item? If two items cost the same, but one is of higher quality, we buy the item of higher quality. The same goes for health care, but there are some complexities. Some of these complexities are driving the current debate.

Using the equation, if we wish to maximize value, we should maximize quality and decrease costs (somewhat cynically, this is what the purchasers of health care want), or we could increase quality without increasing costs (this is what the recipients of the purchased health care want). Realistically, however, society wants the highest possible quality at a reasonable price.

Cost containment was clearly the initial driving force behind managed care. It is obvious that, to succeed, the industry will have to move beyond mere cost cutting. Moreover, the cost-cutting phenomena will soon dissipate. There will come a point when networks, practices, and physicians will no longer be able to compete on price. At that point, all unnecessary or discretionary expenses will have been removed and systems will have to compete on quality—first on quality of service and then, more important, on quality of care. Most feel this is where the competition should have been focused all along.

Achieving, Maintaining, and Improving Quality

Once quality has been assessed and measured, there are two basic approaches to achieving, maintaining, and improving quality: quality assurance and quality improvement. Quality assurance (QA) describes the standard quality assurance and quality control procedures that many equate with a quality management program. Fortunately, quality is much more. In discussing quality improvement (QI), commonly used terms include total quality management (TQM) and continuous quality improvement (CQI). TQM is primarily a managerial style, and CQI is a series of tools and methods used in improving quality.

QA is a "formal and systematic exercise in identifying problems in medical care delivery, designing activities to overcome the problems, and carrying out follow-up monitoring to ensure that no new problems have been introduced and that corrective steps have been effective."[9]

QA is an inspection process, i.e., looking for the bad apple, a search and destroy management style. The basis for QA is chart audits or reviews. QA methods attempt to determine whether what is recorded in the medical record is appropriate care for that patient. For example, nurses, physicians, or other personnel review charts, checking for inappropriately managed hypertension, an elevated blood sugar, or an overlooked or abnormal laboratory test. In other situations, an event—such as unplanned admission, death in the hospital, procedural complication, or readmission to the ICU—triggers a review. QA looks for blame.

It is safe to say that physicians are not fond of QA programs, and studies have shown that QA has not been a particularly effective tool for improving quality. These activities are seen as consuming an inordinate amount of time, producing little or no new information, and too often leading to punitive action.[2]

Quality assurance programs are necessary but are not sufficient. Most of us are not incompetent or criminal, but all of us could do things better. That is where quality improvement (TQM, CQI) becomes valuable. Quality improvement is "a set of techniques for continuous study and improvement of the process of delivering health care services and products to meet the needs and expectations of the customers of those services and products."[1]

Total Quality Management

Quality improvement, in the form of TQM, was introduced in Japan by W. Edwards Deming shortly after WW II. TQM is widely felt to be the catalyst for turning the image of Japanese products from "junk" to the high-quality perception of today. TQM was introduced into U.S. manufacturing in the 1970s and into the health care industry in the mid- to late 1980s. TQM is a process, a program, a set of tools. Perhaps more important, it is a philosophy. It is the driving force of the organization that fosters a cycle of never-ending improvement (i.e., CQI). It is the relentless pursuit of excellence.

TQM seeks to constantly improve the work being done and to eliminate errors and mistakes by doing it right the first time. The goal is no unnecessary complexity, no waste, minimal inspection, no rework, and no recalls. There is an emphasis on "zero defects." Philip Crosby has stated that, "Quality is Free."[5] What becomes costly is not doing things right the first time. Total quality management is a systematic way of guaranteeing that things happen the way they were planned.

There are three key principles of TQM: customer focus, management by data, and process improvement. TQM suggests that you seek customer satisfaction by adopting a customer-centered approach. The patient is the customer, of course, but internal customers should not be forgotten. Internal customers are those within your organization who are affected in some way by your work. Remember that the job of every worker involves being a customer, a processor, and a supplier. It is vital that you strive to meet and exceed the expectations of your customers.

TQM insists that you manage by using data (i.e., manage by facts). TQM stresses the use of scientific method instead of intuition to solve problems. Do not manage by anecdote, and remember that quality is measurable. Use the same scientific method employed in research to evaluate and monitor quality standards. Based on the data, find out where you have a problem and fix it.

Finally, improve the process by which work is accomplished. Assume that employees want to do a good job. Most problems or defects arise from bad processes, not bad people. It has been estimated that 15 percent of errors are due to people and that 85 percent are due to inefficiencies in processes.[10]

Therefore, focus on improving processes. The basic method by which processes are improved is teamwork (multidisciplinary and cross-functional teams). TQM suggests that those who do the work know best how to do it better. Managers merely empower and coach employees. The key is to improve the process by which work is accomplished and to reduce process variation. Both actions combine to improve outcomes.

QA vs. QI

A comparison of QA and QI highlights the differences.[11] QA seeks to eliminate the lower "tail" of the statistical distribution. The focus is on outliers. QA is primarily a retrospective inspection process. The focus is on correcting problems after they have occurred, rather than preventing them. Problems are identified after the fact, and individuals are found at fault. The spotlight is on the perpetrator and what he or she did or did not do. QI, on the other hand, seeks to improve the mean. QI seeks to raise the "average" performance (i.e., move the whole curve). The target is processes, not individuals. Outliers must still be investigated, but overall quality will have improved.

Quality assurance is necessary. Quality improvement, utilizing total quality management and continuous quality improvement techniques, supplements QA efforts to form a more effective quality management program.

The Importance of Total Quality Improvement

American medicine is acknowledged to be the best in the world. It's not the cheapest, but I think most people in the world would rather be in the United States if they were sick or injured. Of course, that is the individual's point of view. If you look at group measures of health, the United States doesn't come out on top. Our life expectancy is not ranked first. We also rank amazingly low in infant mortality rates. There are many reasons for these results. Still, we could be doing better.

We need to make health care in the United States more cost effective (i.e., contain costs) and more patient friendly (i.e., improve the quality of service), and we need to improve outcomes (i.e., improve the quality of care). The bottom line is that we need to improve the total quality of U.S. health care. To do so, cost containment, quality of service, and quality of care must be given equal emphasis. You can't compromise quality to save money, but, given limited resources, the cost of what we do must be considered.

Efforts to improve the total quality of health care in the United States have gathered public support and momentum. Unfortunately, physicians have been skeptical of the many new quality initiatives that are being discussed and implemented.[12] One reason may be that some of these initiatives grew out of efforts to reduce costs through the use of managed care. The intent of the initiatives seems to be to direct physicians to use fewer resources, rather than to improve the quality of care. In this way, quality initiatives are seen by physicians as thinly veiled attempts to cut costs. Another reason is the intimidation factor. Some of these initiatives involve summarizing a physician's patient care, comparing it to other physicians, and even making the comparisons public. Report cards have always engendered anxiety. Finally, there is the perception that we've seen it all before. In the past, efforts to assure quality have not, in fact, been particularly effective in improving quality. These activities have been seen as consuming an inordinate amount of time, producing little or no new information, and often leading to punitive actions.[2]

As a result, clinicians have been wary and defensive about quality data, their collection, and their interpretation. Physicians must recognize, however, that the goal of these quality initiatives is to improve patient care and that new processes are being put in place to bring about this goal without the onerous, "Big Brother," punitive programs of the past.

Blumenthal has stated that: "Although it is understandable that so many physicians have reacted to the debate over the quality of care with anger, skepticism, or simply disinterest, such reactions are a luxury that physicians can no longer afford. Physicians owe it to themselves and their patients to master the substantive issues that underlie current discussions about the quality of care."[6]

Outcomes Research and Management

Outcomes are those changes, either adverse or favorable, in the actual or potential health status of persons, groups, or communities that can be attributed to prior or concurrent care.[7] Until recently, outcomes were measured in clinical terms, such as longevity, morbidity, mortality, complications, and physical functioning. Outcomes recently have been expanded to include measures of psychological functioning, quality of life, resource utilization, cost of care, and satisfaction.[13]

Research into the outcomes of health care delivery is the investigation of the value of health care interventions. The basic intent is to measure the success of a specific procedure or treatment from the patient's point of view. Because the goal of medical care for most patients is to obtain a more effective life and to preserve functioning and well-being, the patient is in the best position to judge the outcome. In this vein, outcomes research is based on patient satisfaction or perception.

Although conceptually similar, outcomes research is different from clinical research. Clinical research is conducted to determine the efficacy of a treatment under controlled study conditions. Efficacy is the probability of benefit to individuals in a defined population from a medical technology applied for a given medical problem under ideal conditions of use.[14] Efficacy answers the question: Does the treatment work? Outcomes research is concerned with the effectiveness and efficiency of the treatment. Effectiveness is the probability of benefit to individuals in a defined population from a medical technology applied for a given medical problem under average conditions of use.[14] Effectiveness answers the question: Does the treatment work in actual practice? Efficiency is the degree of quality present in a given unit of health care for which a fixed amount of resources is used.[14] Efficiency answers the question: Is the treatment worth its costs?[13]

In outcomes research, costs, patient satisfaction, and quality of life are measured. Costs are also termed "economic outcomes." One can apply the new science of medical economics and derive such functions as cost identification, cost-benefit analysis, and cost effectiveness. Patient satisfaction is the prime example of less tangible results often categorized as "societal outcomes." Patient satisfaction is measured by questionnaire or survey, complaints and complaint rates, health plan re-enrollment rates, and contract renewals.. Quality of life is also termed "health outcomes." Quality of life is usually measured by questionnaire or survey.

It is not enough simply to measure outcomes in the delivery of health care; we must do something with the data, and that is where outcomes management comes into play. Outcomes studies provide the answer to the question, "How am I doing?" By benchmarking, you can compare your outcomes to those of others. Benchmarking is the process of measuring a characteristic of your organization against the same characteristic of another organization known for its quality.[15] If you do not compare favorably, find out why and change. If you compare favorably, use the results for marketing.

Clinical Practice Guidelines, Parameters, Pathways, Protocols, Algorithms

There are subtle differences among the terms, but clinical practice guidelines (CPGs), parameters, pathways, protocols, and algorithms are basically all variations on a theme. These are statements systematically developed to assist practitioners and patients in their decisions about care for specific clinical circumstances.[16] Guidelines help to ensure that the technical process of care is guided by scientifically sound, best practices.[13] The push for CPGs grew out of research showing large variations in practices.

For example, in one county in Maine, 70 percent of women had had a hysterectomy by age 70. In a nearby county, only 20 percent of such women had had this procedure.[17] From these findings, one can deduce either that unnecessary care is sometimes being provided or that necessary care is being withheld.

Practice guidelines or parameters are constructed by gathering all available information about a patient care problem, evaluating how best to manage that problem in light of that knowledge, and using that knowledge to create a guideline that can assist physicians in the management of that problem.[12] At their best, practice guidelines are "evidence-based medicine" (i.e., they are based on solid published research).

Positive aspects of CPGs include standard accepted evidence-based algorithms, incorporation of "best practices," and excellent educational tools. Physicians may not be aware of best practices because of gaps in training, limited experience, or insufficient time or motivation. Guidelines may be beneficial in promulgating new information. Their use also may provide some protection from medical liability.

Negative aspects of CPGs include concern over creating "cookbook" medicine and opening up liability problems if guidelines are not followed. There is insufficient scientific evidence for many things physicians do. In these cases, expert opinion and consensus are relied upon to construct the guideline. But the consensus may be wrong, and the status quo may be legitimized as fact when it may not be correct. For many situations, clinical practice guidelines just aren't applicable—for example, where the problem does not fit into a clear and simple diagnostic category, or where two or three things are going on simultaneously. Finally, the patient may not want the treatment suggested by the guideline.

THE BUSINESS SIDE OF MEDICINE:
A Survival Primer for Medical Students and Residents

Utilization Review and Management

Utilization review and management involve surveillance of and intervention into the clinical activities of physicians for the purpose of controlling costs, such actions as precertification for hospitalizations and procedures, concurrent review of hospitalized patients, and use of case managers.[18]

Utilization management (UM) focuses on efficient treatment (i.e., critical pathways), appropriate level of care, and appropriate length of care. UM seeks to influence physician behavior.[18] The mechanism is simple and direct (denial of payment for services deemed unnecessary).[18]

UM is performed by the organization at financial risk. Under fee for service, it is the insurance companies. Under diagnosis-related groups (DRGs) , it is the hospital. Under capitation contracts, it is the group practice. UM, however, may become micromanagement at its worst by inserting an administrative hassle into the physician-patient relationship. UM may actually cost more money than it saves. To avoid some of the onerous features of UM, several other approaches have been taken.

Practice profiling uses summary data on practice patterns and identifies physicians whose overall, rather than individual, use of services deviates from the standard of other physicians in the community. Outliers are then subject to various interventions. Profiling may be used for initial selection, deselection, recredentialing, education, sanctions, and rewards. A special type of profiling is termed economic profiling (or economic credentialing). Some MCOs offer contracts only to those physicians whose practice patterns are in accord with the plan's cost-control objectives.

Accreditation and Accrediting bodies

The Joint Commission on Accreditation of Healthcare Organizations (JCAHO) is the body that accredits hospitals. Accreditation by JCAHO provides "deemed status" for federal programs. Such status is necessary to receive federal money. JCAHO has recently expanded the scope of its accreditation activities beyond the inpatient hospital arena to ambulatory clinics and behavioral health programs.

The National Committee for Quality Assurance (NCQA) offers accreditation for managed care organizations (MCOs) NCQA was founded in 1979 by two managed care trade associations, the American Managed Care and Review Association and the Group Health Association of America. Responding to concerns about the quality of and access to care in some of the early HMOs, these organizations came to the conclusion that the managed care industry must develop standards and be accountable for them, or risk oversight by a plethora of government agencies. NCQA soon became independent of its founders and grew when the employer community took an active leadership role in the organization.[19] NCQA has become the informal standard for accrediting MCOs. NCQA accreditation is not necessary for MCO operation, but obtaining such a designation offers a distinct marketing advantage.

NCQA accreditation focuses on six areas:

- Quality improvement (a well-organized, comprehensive quality improvement program accountable to the organization's highest levels).

- Credentialing (review of a practitioner's credentials for the purpose of determining if criteria for clinical privileging are met and ensuring that members are served by qualified providers).

- Utilization management (evidence that the UM program does not serve as a barrier to appropriate care).

- Patient's rights and responsibilities (evidence of a commitment to patient rights and of mechanisms to protect and enhance patient satisfaction with services).

- Preventive health services (focus on prevention and early detection).

- Medical records (records reviewed to ensure high-quality documentation of quality of care).

Performance Measurement by Report Cards

In the past, it was assumed that physicians delivered high-quality care. Quality was rarely questioned and rarely measured. Purchasers of health care usually just paid what the physician billed, assuming the patient was receiving the highest quality care. This was before cost became the driving force. Now, purchasers (whether individual patients, employers, or insurance companies) will not automatically pay what is billed. Purchasers want the most for their money. They want proof that they are getting their money's worth. Report cards provide purchasers of care with information to decide whether to continue seeking care from institutions and/or providers. The subject of the report card could be the individual physician, the group practice, or the health plan.

The Health Plan Employer Data and Information Set (HEDIS) is an example of a report card for managed care health plans. HEDIS originally included 28 performance standards, such as hospital days per thousand enrollees, rates of retinal screening for diabetes, rates of cholesterol screening, and mammography rates. The latest version contains more than 60 performance measures.

Some type of score card, or report card, on health plans is likely to prove to be an enduring feature of our new health system. Influential groups, such as the federal

THE BUSINESS SIDE OF MEDICINE:
A Survival Primer for Medical Students and Residents

government and business, believe that such data are needed for an informed choice in the purchase of care. Individual consumers seem to strongly support the release of data on performance of individual practitioners. The release of malpractice data via the Internet in Florida is an example. Pennsylvania and New York have compiled and released annual statistics on mortality after CABG surgeries for individual surgeons and hospitals. Look for expansion of this type of publicly available data.

As you might imagine, there are many problems with report cards. Risk adjustment is a major obstacle. If you handle all the tough cases or see the sickest patients, you are going to look bad. In addition, most report cards now measure processes rather than outcomes. Outcomes are really what the public wants. Much work needs to be done to make these "report cards" optimally useful. Report cards, however, are not going to go away

The Physician's Role

Physicians need to overcome some of their resistance to accountability to nonphysicians (administrators, government, consumers).[20] Accountability is a reality. I want my plumber to be held accountable for his or her work. Why not physicians? Physicians need to form working alliances with these powerful groups. To cooperate, physicians need to develop the behavioral skills required to function in interdisciplinary teams. Skills, such as leadership, team-building, and negotiating, are important. Some of these skills are not ingrained in some physicians. They have to be learned. Physicians need to show leadership in assessing and improving the quality of care. They need to develop a reasonable degree of sophistication with methods and tools used to assess and measure quality and a critical appreciation of their strengths and weaknesses. Finally, physicians must be advocates for individual patients. They must temper the drive toward cost containment where quality is compromised. It is possible and likely that high-quality care costs less. Make no mistake, however; quality is the prime directive for physicians.

References

1. Institute of Medicine. Medicare: *A Strategy for Quality Assurance*. Washington, D.C.: National Academy Press, 1990.

2. Barbour, G. "Assuring Quality in the Department of Veterans Affairs: What Can the Private Sector Learn?" *Journal of Clinical Outcomes Management* 2(5):67-76, Sept.-Oct. 1995.

3. "The Quality Imperative." *Fortune* 114(7), March 21, 1988.

4. Soper, M., and others. Balancing the Triad: *Cost Containment, Quality of Service and Quality of Care in Managed Care Systems*. Kansas City, Mo.: National Center

for Managed Health Care Administration, 1990.

5. Crosby, P. *Quality Is Free*. New York, N.Y.: New American Library, 1979.

6. Blumenthal, D. "Quality of Care—What Is It?" *New England Journal of Medicine* 335(12):891-4, Sept. 19, 1996.

7. Donabedian A. *Explorations in Quality Assessment and Monitoring*. Ann Arbor, Mich.: Health Administration Press, 1980.

8. Berwick, D., and others. *Curing Health Care*. San Francisco, Calif.: Jossey-Bass, Inc., 1990.

9. Lohr, K., and Brook, R. "Quality Assurance in Medicine." *American Behavioral Scientist* 27(5):583-607, March 1984.

10. Gryna, F., and Juran, J. *Juran's Quality Control Handbook*, 4th Ed. New York, N.Y.: McGraw-Hill, 1988.

11. Baslestracci, D., and Barlow, J. Quality Improvement. *Practical Applications for Medical Group Practice*. Englewood, Colo.: Center for Research in Ambulatory Health Care Administration, 1994.

12. Goldfield, N., and Nash, D. *The Challenge of Improving Quality*. Chicago, Ill.: American Medical Association, 1994.

13. "IMCARE Quality 101." Philadelphia, Pa.: American Society of Internal Medicine, 1998.

14. *Putting Research to Work in Quality Improvement and Quality Assurance*. Publication No. 93-0034. Washington, D.C.: Agency for Health Care Policy and Research, Public Health Service, Department of Health and Human Services, 1993.

15. Gaucher, E., and Coffey, R. *Total Quality in Health Care*. San Francisco, Calif.: Jossey-Bass, 1993.

16. Institute of Medicine. *Guidelines for Clinical Practice: From Development to Use. Washington*, D.C.: National Academy Press, 1992.

17. Wennberg, J. "Dealing with Medical Practice Variations: A Proposal for Action." *Health Affairs* 3(2):3-32, Summer 1984.

18. Bodenheimer, T., and Grumbach, K. *Understanding Health Policy: A Clinical Approach.* Stamford, Conn.: Appleton & Lange, 1995.

19. Rosenberg, R. *Demonstrating Quality and Efficiency in Managed Care Organizations.* Chicago, Ill.: American Medical Association, 1994.

20. DesHarnais, S., and McLaughlin, C. "Clinical Quality, Risk-Adjustment, and Outcomes Measured in Academic Health Centers." In *Managing in an Academic Health Care Environment,* Minogue, W., Editor. Tampa, Fla.: American College of Physician Executives, 1992.

W. Michael Alberts, MD, MBA, is Professor and Associate Chair, Department of Internal Medicine, and Medical Director of Quality Management, University of South Florida Physicians Group, Tampa, Florida.

CHAPTER 6

Legal Environment of Medicine
by Bryan Burgess, JD, MPH

This chapter is a synopsis of the legal environment in which physicians practice their profession. The goal is to orient physicians, especially those beginning their careers, to selected legal topics that pertain to physicians' decision making and actions in the clinical setting and in the commercial arena. In recognition of the jurisdictional, temporal, and interpretive variability and complexity of law, this chapter will provide only generalized information intended to:

- Heighten the sensitivity of physicians to assorted legal responsibilities, rights, risks, and liabilities that are inherent in their profession.

- Stimulate a precautionary approach and further inquiry by the physician encountering a situation or a transaction posing legally significant issues and consequences.

The subjects to be covered in this chapter include an overview of the legal system; physicians' licensure, discipline, and employment status; physicians' relationship with patients; physicians' relationship with payers; physicians' relationship with other physicians and other health care providers; and other regulatory considerations.

The Legal System

Preliminary to a review of specific legal topics, it is important to provide a brief overview of the government institutions and system by which the law is formulated and applied. The United States consists of both federal and state governments, each of which has its own constitutions and legislative, executive, and judicial branches. The conventional rendering of the roles of these institutions is that the legislative branch (i.e., Congress at the federal level and the legislatures at the state level) makes the law; the executive branch (i.e., the President and federal agencies at the federal level and the governors and state agencies at the state level) enforces the law; and the judicial branch (i.e., the various courts at the local, state, and federal levels) interprets the law.

Under the "federalism" established by the U.S. Constitution, the states have collectively ceded certain powers to the federal government and have otherwise retained their own governments and systems of laws. The federal government's authority has been construed very broadly, to the effect that Congress may enact laws affecting any activity involving "interstate commerce" or the "public welfare" (assuming federal funds are involved). Thus, under its public welfare authority, the federal government has created programs, such as Medicare and Medicaid, that have had a significant impact on physicians. Based on its authority to regulate interstate commerce, the federal government has passed legislation, such as the various antitrust laws, affecting the business practices of physicians.

The federal regulatory approach to health care has evolved through several phases over the years. From the 1940s through the 1970s, federal laws focused on promoting the development of health care resources. For example, the Hill-Burton Act in 1942 initiated a federal-state program of hospital planning and construction, and the Health Professions Educational Assistance Act in 1963 authorized a program of direct federal aid to medical and health professional schools and students. In the mid-1970s, the emphasis shifted to controlling health care facility development. The National Health Planning and Resource Development Act of 1974 assigned health planning responsibilities to state and local agencies and required a "certificate of need" from the state for health facility development and expansion. Since enactment of Medicare and Medicaid in 1965, various initiatives have attempted to ensure high-quality care and to control costs in these programs (such as the shift in 1983 from a retrospective, cost-based reimbursement system for hospital services to prospectively determined payment rates based on diagnosis-related groups (DRGs), and the change in 1992 to a Medicare Fee Schedule for physician payment). Dramatic reforms to address access and cost concerns were debated and rejected in 1993-94. Of interest to physicians, in recent years the federal government moved to control costs through an emphasis on policy and enforcement initiatives to prevent overutilization and fraud.

As a consequence of federalism, the states have primary authority over most legal subjects of concern to physicians: licensure, discipline, tort law (including medical malpractice), contract law, employment law, insurance regulation, confidentiality, and other patient rights.

There are some areas in which federal and state laws may overlap. In some instances, federal laws preempt the substantive area they address to the exclusion of state law. This preemption doctrine is intended to promote a unified approach to issues deemed nationally significant. For example, the Employment Retirement Income Security Act of 1974 (ERISA),[1] establishes uniform national standards for employee benefits plans and broadly preempts state laws attempting to regulate such plans. Therefore, for example, a patient's legal challenge to a self-funded employer health plan's decision to deny coverage of particular medical services must be brought in federal court and reviewed under the terms of ERISA, notwithstanding any state laws.

The U.S. Constitution establishes the parameters within which federal and state governments may develop other laws and rules. In addition, the states are circumscribed by their respective state constitutions. The laws that legislatures pass are usually called "statutes." The legislative branch frequently delegates authority to administrative agencies in the executive branch to make "rules" or "regulations" to address specific issues and situations under a general statutory framework. These administrative agencies are also frequently authorized to establish their own "judicial" bodies to decide disputes arising under the agency's rules. It is normally necessary to exhaust these administrative review procedures before the matter may be considered by a court.

At the federal level, several agencies have jurisdiction over health care-related matters. The Department of Health and Human Services (HHS), and the Health Care Financing Administration (HCFA) within HHS, have administrative and rule-making responsibility for the Medicare and the Medicaid programs. The HHS Office of Inspector General (OIG) has enforcement responsibility for these programs. The U.S. Department of Justice (DOJ) and the Federal Trade Commission (FTC) have responsibility for enforcement of the federal antitrust laws. The Internal Revenue Service (IRS), within the U.S. Department of Treasury, has administrative and rule-making responsibility for tax-related issues affecting the health care industry.

At the state level, agencies with various names (departments of health, professional regulation, etc.) have jurisdiction over regulation and licensure of health professionals and facilities. The states typically have commissioners or departments of insurance with jurisdiction over the business of insurance, including health insurance and health maintenance organizations. The states' attorneys general normally have authority to enforce state antitrust and criminal statutes pertinent to health care. The responsibility to regulate the state aspects of the Medicaid program is usually delegated to a state social services or health agency.

The judicial system has responsibility for interpreting and applying the law at the federal and state levels. Interpretation by courts occurs through decision making in individual cases that present particular legal questions. Courts' decisions reflecting their holdings and reasoning in cases are recorded in books called "reporters." The U.S. Supreme Court and the lower federal courts have authority to review all federal laws to determine their constitutionality and meaning and, in the case of federal administrative agency regulations, whether they are within the scope of authority delegated by Congress. The federal courts also have authority to review the validity, under the U.S. Constitution, of any state constitutional, statutory, or regulatory provision. State courts have ultimate authority to determine the meaning of state laws. By virtue of this interpretive function, courts have the opportunity to "make" law. At times, the courts develop legal principles to govern the cases they are deciding. This court-made law is called the "common law." In areas of civil law, such as contract law and tort law, many of the guiding principles are based on common law rather than on statutes or regulations. Under the doctrine of *stare decisis*, courts resolve present controversies by following common law principles or precedents established in past cases.

Licensure and Discipline

By virtue of their inherent power to protect the public health, safety, and welfare, the states have jurisdiction to regulate the practice of medicine and individuals engaging in this profession. In all of the states, legislatures have enacted medical practice laws intended to ensure that individuals engaged in the practice of medicine in the state meet certain minimum requirements and observe certain standards of conduct. Individuals who fall below these requirements, or who violate these standards, may be disciplined or barred from practice in the state. The various state legislatures enact laws to establish the general parameters and to delegate specific regulatory powers and duties to administrative agencies (such as a department of professional regulation, a board of medicine, etc.).

The foremost regulation is the requirement that every person desiring to practice medicine must first obtain a license to do so from the state, unless a statutory exemption applies. State laws may specify exemptions from licensure, such as for licensed physicians from another state or country who are only consulting with a licensed physician in the state; commissioned medical officers of the U.S. armed forces and the Public Health Service, while on activity duty; and residents and interns in approved training programs who are registered with the state and/or meet other specified conditions. State laws may also provide for limited licenses and temporary permits for individuals to practice in narrowly prescribed circumstances. The state law normally specifies a period for which the medical license is effective and provides that the license will revert to inactive status unless the renewal application and applicable fee are submitted on a timely basis. A physician whose license becomes inactive must cease practicing medicine until the license is reactivated.

The state's laws prescribe the qualifications to be demonstrated by applicants as a condition for licensure. The details of such requirements vary but include educational standards and character standards. The procedures for obtaining a license are defined by statute and rule and generally require a person desiring to be licensed to apply to the designated administrative agency and make the necessary showing of qualifications and competence. This typically includes passing the state's designated examination. Currently, state laws generally designate the licensure examination of the Federation of State Medical Boards of the U.S, Inc., (FLEX) or the U.S. Medical Licensing Examination (USMLE). Because the license to practice medicine is a valuable property right that cannot be denied arbitrarily, or for unlawful reasons, the decision of the licensing agency is subject to appeal for further administrative and/or judicial review.

The states' legislatures delegate to administrative agencies the authority to discipline licensed physicians based on determinations that cause, as defined by statute and/or rule, exists for such actions. Such disciplinary actions may include revocation, suspension, or denial of renewal of the license; restriction of scope of practice; public or private reprimand or censure; civil monetary penalty; and probation, with conditions such as treatment, continuing medical education, reexamination, or supervision by another physician.

The states' laws specify a great number and variety of standards of conduct, violation of which is grounds for disciplinary action. Physicians should familiarize themselves with these standards in the states in which they are licensed. Examples of such standards and grounds for disciplinary action include:

- Making of misrepresentations in the application for license or renewal, or in other records or reports.

- Conviction for a crime related to the practice of medicine or the ability to practice medicine.

- Having a license to practice in another state acted against by that state's licensing agency.

- False or misleading advertising.

- Advertising or practicing under another name.

- Failing to report to the state's licensing agency any person who the physician knows is in violation of the state's medical practice laws and rules.

- Failing to perform any statutory or legal obligation imposed on licensed physicians, including failing to file any report or record required by state or federal law.

- Exercising influence within a patient-physician relationship for the purpose of sexual activity (generally, a patient is presumed to be incapable of giving free informed consent to sexual activity with his or her physician).

- Soliciting patients, either personally or through an agent, through the use of fraud or undue influence.

- Failing to keep written medical records justifying a course of treatment.

- Exercising influence on the patient for the financial gain of the physician or of a third party, including promoting or selling of services, goods, appliances, or drugs.

- Performing professional services without patient consent, except as otherwise permitted by law.

- Prescribing or dispensing drugs or controlled substances other than in the course of the physician's professional practice, or prescribing or dispensing drugs or controlled substances inappropriately or in excessive quantities.

- Prescribing or dispensing certain controlled drugs to him- or herself.

- Being unable to practice medicine with reasonable skill and safety to patients by reason of illness, use of drugs or alcohol, or other mental or physical condition.

- Gross or repeated malpractice.

- Performing services beyond the scope of competence.

- Delegating professional responsibility to a person who the physician knows or has reason to know is not qualified by training, experience, or license.

- Failing to adequately supervise nurses, physician assistants, and others acting under the physician's supervision.

- Pre-signing blank prescription forms.

- Paying or receiving any commission, bonus, kickback, or rebate, or engaging in any split-fee arrangement in any form with a physician, organization, or person, either directly or indirectly, for patients referred to providers of health care goods and services.

The state's designated agency must follow procedures prescribed by statute in disciplining a licensed physician. The state's statutes usually allow the filing of complaints against physicians by patients and others alleging violations of the laws and rules governing the profession. The procedures for handling such complaints normally provide for a preliminary investigation and "probable cause" determination and may confer confidentiality during this initial phase. The physician will be notified of this investigation and of the substance of the complaint, unless it is determined that such notification would be detrimental to the investigation or unless the act under investigation is a crime. It is advisable for a physician to retain an attorney as soon as he or she knows that an investigation has been initiated and prior to any written or verbal communications with the investigators.

If the agency's investigative staff and/or review panel determines that probable cause exists, a formal complaint may be filed and prosecuted against the physician. In this circumstance, the physician will be given notice of the charge and of the facts on which it is based and an opportunity to appear and make a defense at formal disciplinary proceedings. The states' laws frequently provide for an emergency proceeding for the suspension of the license of a physician who presents dangers to the public. Such proceedings will be more abbreviated than those required for a final license revocation or other discipline. The state law may provide for a hearing officer to conduct a formal hearing or may designate a quasi-judicial agency board to hear evidence and resolve the issues. The state law will also provide the physician with a right to seek judicial review of the action and order of the regulatory agency.

The laws in many states are evolving to recognize consumer interest in information about health care providers. They are requiring physicians to provide extensive data pertaining to their education, professional experience, malpractice claims experience, disciplinary actions by licensing agencies and hospital medical staffs, and other such information for publication via the Internet and by other means.

Employment Status

Approximately 75 percent of physicians will practice their profession as employees of organizations, such as group practices, hospitals, physician practice management companies, health maintenance organizations, or medical schools. The physician's employment relationship and associated legal rights and obligations will invariably be based on and defined by a written employment contract and other organizational policies and documents that may be incorporated by reference in the contract. Contract terms and conditions will usually extend beyond the obvious issues of compensation and benefits, assigned duties, and term of commitment and will include various matters with profound implications for the physician's interests both during and subsequent to the employment relationship. A few examples of such matters include:

- The employer's furnishing of medical malpractice insurance with adequate financial limits and "tail coverage" for the physician for claims made after the physician departs from the employment relationship.

- Non-competition covenants restricting the physician's ability to practice or consult outside the employment relationship and to practice within a defined market area for a specified period following the end of employment.

- Provisions concerning the employer's ownership and control of patient and business information and intellectual property created by the physician.

- Provisions concerning confidentiality and non-use of information.

- Provisions subjecting the physician to financial obligations and penalties.

It is not uncommon for physicians, particularly those beginning their careers, to sign such employment contracts without question, assuming them to be archetypal and immutable. However, physicians should be cognizant of the potential legal complexities and perils that may be presented by employment contracts and proceed with commensurate caution, ideally including competent legal review and advice.

THE BUSINESS SIDE OF MEDICINE:
A Survival Primer for Medical Students and Residents

Physician's Relationship with Patients

Creation and Termination of Relationship

In the absence of a preexisting contract with a party, such as a hospital or a managed care organization, obligating the physician to accept and provide care to a patient, the general rule is that a physician is free to decline to establish a professional relationship with an individual. However, once a physician has agreed, expressly or by implication, to accept a patient, the physician-patient relationship imposes certain duties on the physician, such as the duty of care and the duty not to abandon treatment. Physicians should be mindful that the physician-patient relationship is not necessarily predicated on an express or detailed agreement. It may be implied from the physician's conduct, such as a telephone call or "off-hours" conversation in which the physician is informed of an individual's medical condition and provides medical advice. When a physician-patient relationship is created, the physician will be responsible for providing care until the relationship is ended in an appropriate manner. The relationship can be terminated by the physician for various reasons, including the patient's noncompliance or nonpayment, provided that the physician gives reasonable advance notice to the patient. This notice should be in writing, with proof of delivery; suggest other qualified physicians for the patient's condition; offer to transfer copies of medical records to the patient's new physician; and offer availability to provide care for a specified reasonable period (e.g., 10 days) while the patient makes alternative arrangements. Termination of the relationship with a hospitalized patient must be accomplished in accordance with the hospital's medical staff bylaws and policies. If the patient has withdrawn from or terminated the physician's care, it is advisable for the physician to send a letter to the patient to document the end of the relationship.

Consent

The physician must obtain the patient's consent prior to treatment. This duty to obtain consent is recognized by common law, many state statutes, and the standards of the Joint Commission on Accreditation of Healthcare Organizations (JCAHO). Failure to obtain consent may result in tort claims for battery and negligence. It is not necessary for the patient's consent to be direct and explicit, and the physician may rely on implied consent for routine medical treatment with minimal risk. Because of the physician's potential liability for failure to obtain informed consent, it is advisable for the physician to obtain written consent for any treatment or procedure that is complex or involves appreciable risk. It should be noted that, while such a consent document provides important evidence should a question later arise, the essence of the consent process is effective discussion and information-sharing between the physician and the patient. The physician should include a note regarding the consent discussion as well as the signed consent form in the patient's medical record.

In the absence of a statute authorizing delegation, the physician who will perform the treatment or procedure has personal responsibility to obtain consent and should not delegate the task to nurses, residents, or other personnel. The physician should use language that is understandable by the patient and may supplement the discussion with visual aids and literature. In general, the patient should be given a clear and concise explanation of the nature of his or her condition, the nature and purpose of the treatment, alternatives to the proposed treatment, the risks of no treatment, and information about the physician's pertinent experience and ability. Where applicable, the patient should be informed of the identity and status of other health care personnel who will have significant responsibility in performing the treatment.

The patient should have the opportunity to ask questions. The consent discussion must occur at a time when the patient is not sedated or otherwise impaired, and the patient should be afforded as much time as is needed to reflect on the information and to make a decision. The presence of witnesses is advisable where the patient's condition or the treatment risks are unusual. If the patient has been determined by a court to be legally incompetent, or if the physician determines that the patient lacks the capacity for understanding and decision making, consent should be obtained from a third party. This party may be a court-appointed guardian, a surrogate designated by the patient in accordance with state law allowing such a health care proxy, a family member, or other persons as may be defined by state statute. If the patient is a non-emancipated minor, the physician should obtain consent from the minor's parents or guardian, unless state law provides an exception (such as for an emergency, sexually transmitted diseases, abortion, etc.) For hospitalized patients, the physician should be aware of and adhere to the hospital's policies and procedures regarding patient consent.

The states have evolved two different standards for evaluating whether there is an adequate level of disclosure by a physician to support a patient's informed consent. The "professional practice" standard, applied in a majority of jurisdictions, requires that the physician disclose all information that a reasonable physician would disclose in similar circumstances. The "reasonable patient" standard adopted in some states requires the physician to disclose all information that a reasonable person in the patient's position would consider "material" in making a decision about the proposed treatment.

There are limited circumstances in which patient consent is not required, such as when a medical emergency must be treated without delay, when the patient requests not to be informed of treatment risks, or when a physician reasonably believes that disclosure would present a serious threat to the patient's health. In addition, when certain unanticipated conditions are discovered during surgery, the physician may proceed to treat that condition if delay or additional surgery would be detrimental to the patient. Most states have laws providing procedures to be followed for involuntary examination and treatment of persons whose mental illness renders them incompetent to consent.

The U.S. Supreme Court has held that a competent person has a constitutionally protected right to refuse unwanted treatment, including life-sustaining medical care.[2] Related to this right is the ability of patients to make advance directives concerning their health care-related decisions, should they lack capacity to express such decisions. The states have varying approaches in terms of the procedural and evidentiary requirements for advance directives, authorizing vehicles such as living wills, durable powers of attorney, and health care surrogates or proxies whereby patients can exercise their right to control the treatment they will receive if they become incompetent.

Physicians who comply with the terms of an advance directive are provided with immunity from liability. However, if there is question about whether an advance directive has been properly executed or is valid in the physician's locale, the physician should obtain legal counsel. A physician who objects to carrying out a patient's advance directive should follow the appropriate steps to terminate the relationship and transfer the patient to the care of another physician. The Patient Self-Determination Act,[3] enacted by Congress in 1990, is intended to ensure that patients are informed of their rights to make health care decisions under applicable state law. The act requires Medicare hospitals, nursing homes, hospices, home health agencies, and HMOs to provide patients, prior to admission or enrollment, written information regarding their right to accept or refuse treatment and to make advance directives. It is advisable for physicians to routinely request information regarding patients' advance directives as a part of the physician's office database.

Medical Records

Patient medical records serve various legal purposes, and the content, maintenance, ownership, and confidentiality of patient medical records are governed by a range of legal rules. Obviously, the principal purpose of medical records is to document patient care and facilitate communication among health care providers. Risk management, quality assurance/peer review programs, and litigation involving the practice of a physician depend on the information contained in medical records. The standards of JCAHO and of the National Committee on Quality Assurance specify in detail the required contents of medical records. Medical records are also critically important for billing and reimbursement purposes. Because of these considerations, it is crucial that medical records be complete, accurate, timely, and legible. Generally speaking, while the specific data elements may vary by state and setting, the medical record will include:

- Personal identification data (name, birth date, gender, marital status, etc.).

- Financial data (employment, health insurance, etc.).

- Social data (family relationships, psychosocial needs).

- Medical data (chief complaint, medical history, results of physical examinations, diagnostic and therapeutic orders, evidence of informed consent, clinical observations, reports of procedures and tests, and results and conclusions after termination of evaluation and treatment).

While the law in most states provides that a patient's medical record is owned by the health care facility or the provider that creates it, it also typically provides that the patient has ownership and control of the information in the record. Thus, the patient generally has the right to consent to or cause transfer of the medical record to another physician or facility and to inspect and copy the record. A physician employed by a medical group or other organization should review his or her employment contract and related organizational policies to determine whether he or she is entitled to receive a list of "his or her" patients and medical records when departing from the employment relationship. Generally, under state law, a medical record is confidential, and access is limited to the patient, the patient's authorized representatives, and health care providers with an interest in the record in connection with the care of the patient. Improper release of medical records may subject a physician to liability for damages to the patient and to sanctions under professional licensure laws.

Both state and federal law define certain exceptions under which patient records may be disclosed without consent. Such exceptions may include release of information to insurance plans and others for billing and reimbursement purposes and to professional licensing bodies and peer review organizations. State and federal laws also establish stricter confidentiality requirements for certain types of medical information. For example, federal law provides special protection for drug and alcohol abuse treatment records, and many states have adopted statutes concerning confidentiality of HIV/AIDS information. Many states have laws that specifically address the medical records of minors, such as providing parents with the right of access and the right to authorize disclosure to others. State laws also may impose the duty on health care providers to report cases of infectious or sexually transmitted disease and HIV/AIDS to the appropriate state health agency. Similarly, state laws frequently require physicians to report to the appropriate state agency information concerning child and elder abuse; births and deaths; gunshot or stab wounds or other injuries occurring during the commission of a crime; and information about blood alcohol level when the patient is suspected of driving under the influence. Federal law requires reporting of certain incidents involving the malfunction of medical devices; certain adverse reactions to transfusions; and death, disability, or illness resulting from administration of any vaccine to a child.

In recent years, there has been growing interest in "electronic medical records," i.e., a computer-based patient record system. Confidentiality laws and requirements apply with equal force to medical records maintained in this medium. It is, therefore, critical to deploy appropriate management and technical safeguards to prevent unauthorized access to and improper disclosure of computerized patient information.

Professional Liability

Professional malpractice liability is probably the most vexing legal matter with which physicians must cope. At a minimum, the risk of a lawsuit by a dissatisfied patient, or another person claiming injury due to the physician, together with financial responsibility requirements imposed by licensure laws and hospital medical staff bylaws, result in the significant cost of malpractice insurance premiums. Because of such liability exposure and legal requirements, it is not realistic or prudent for a physician to "go bare," i.e., practice without malpractice insurance. At worse, a malpractice lawsuit may subject a physician to years of self-examination and time-consuming legal proceedings, as well as the possibility of an adverse outcome that may result in higher insurance premiums, a financially devastating judgment in excess of insurance coverage, and harm to reputation.

The law of medical malpractice is based on theories of fault-based liability. Thus, in the absence of a contract promising a specific result, unless it can be shown that the physician's conduct fell below a level established by law, the patient should not recover damages from the physician simply because the patient suffered an untoward result from treatment. In general, professional liability claims against physicians are predominately based on the tort law of negligence. Negligence may be defined as conduct that falls below the standard established by law for the protection of others against unreasonable risk of harm. In order to recover for negligent malpractice, the party bringing the action (generally known as the "plaintiff") must prove the following elements:

- The existence of the physician's duty to the plaintiff, usually based on the existence of the physician-patient relationship.

- Applicable duty of care and the physician's breach of that duty.

- Compensable injury (e.g., disability, pain and suffering, financial loss) suffered by the plaintiff.

- Legal causation of the plaintiff's injury by the physician's breach of the duty of care.

It should be noted that the physician's intention is not relevant; the culpable acts may be due to inattentiveness, failure of training, inability, or other factors. Generally, the plaintiff has the burden of proving the foregoing elements by a "preponderance of the evidence," which means that the greater weight of the evidence supports the finding. An exception to this rule is the doctrine of *res ipsa loquitur* ("the thing speaks for itself.") According to this doctrine, where an injury is of a kind that does not ordinarily occur in the absence of negligence and was caused by an instrumentality within the control of the physician, the burden of disproving negligence shifts to the defendant. Situations in which this doctrine is applied include, for example, where a surgical sponge is left in the patient's body or the wrong extremity is operated on.

The standard of care against which the physician's conduct is evaluated is usually established by the testimony of medical experts as being what a reasonably prudent practitioner engaged in similar practice would have done under similar circumstances. It should be noted that, in many jurisdictions, if the physician whose negligence is claimed to have created the cause of action is a board-certified specialist or is trained and experienced in a medical specialty, the medical expert who testifies on the standard of care may be a physician who is trained, experienced, and board certified in the same specialty, but who need not be licensed and practicing in the same or a similar community as the defendant physician. This rule may be viewed as establishing a "national" standard of care for specialist physicians.

The standard of care may also be established by reference to the medical literature, hospital policies, accreditation standards, statutes and rules, clinical practice protocols, pharmaceutical instructions and warnings, and the like. It should be noted that the physician is not required to guarantee a successful outcome from treatment and is not held liable for a failure of diagnosis and treatment if it is due to patient variation or to deficiencies in the state of medical knowledge. In addition to the negligence theory, claims in some jurisdictions and cases may be based on the tort law of battery and breach of contract. Battery is an intentional tort in which the essential claim is that the physician's treatment was without or beyond the scope of patient consent. Breach of contract claims rely on the theory that the physician and the patient made an expressed or implied agreement for a particular outcome; this may occur where the physician gives verbal assurances about the effectiveness of treatment. Further, liability may result from defamation; invasion of privacy; vicarious responsibility for nurses and other providers over whom the physician has supervisory responsibility; and, in some jurisdictions, a "failure to warn" persons who may be affected by the patient's condition or treatment.

In many states, reforms have been enacted to control the costs associated with medical malpractice actions and insurance. For example, such laws may require that notice be given a specified time before the lawsuit is commenced and that the notice of claim be supported by the affidavits of medical experts as to violation of the standard of care. It is necessary, in some states, to submit claims for review by medical malpractice mediation panels. Some state laws may place limits on recovery of noneconomic damages and provide for periodic payment of damage awards to cover future expenses.

Physicians can take a number of actions to mitigate their risk of a professional malpractice lawsuit. Of course, it is important for physicians to pursue continuing education and other activities to remain current in their field and be cognizant of the prevailing standard of care. In addition, good communication between the physician and the patient (and the patient's family) has a major role in reducing the physician's exposure to claims. This communication is crucial both prior to treatment, in the context of informed consent and other discussions of the patient's condition and treatment options and risks, and post-treatment when there has been an adverse occurrence or outcome. The physician's accessibility and sensitivity following an untoward event can be a significant factor in whether the patient decides to make a claim.

In this regard, the physician should carefully review any delinquent patient account before referring it to a collection agency or an attorney. Physicians should be mindful of the potential value of a witness for certain patient consultations and should remember the advice, "If it's not in the medical record, it didn't happen." In addition to the importance of accurate and complete medical records in ensuring high quality in the ongoing care of patients, such records are essential to reconstruction of events in connection with a claim or a lawsuit. Finally, physicians should promptly notify their insurance carrier and consult with legal counsel when there has been a maloccurence or another indication of a potential claim, such as an attorney's request for medical records.

Physician's Relationship with Payers

Federal Fraud and Abuse and Self-Referral Laws

This section discusses two areas of federal law that are important to physicians who accept payment from Medicare or Medicaid:

- Fraud and abuse laws.

- Self-referral prohibition laws.

The federal fraud and abuse laws prohibit various corrupt activities that result in waste of government funds under the Medicare and Medicaid programs. Generally, these laws, commonly referred to as the Anti-Kickback Law,[4] prohibit knowing and willful offering or making of payment, or solicitation or receipt of anything of value, to induce a referral of a patient for items or services for which payment may be made, in whole or in part, by the Medicare or the Medicaid programs. It should be noted that many states have enacted laws that extend the kickback prohibition to all referrals (including non-Medicare/non-Medicaid patients). Violation of the federal Anti-Kickback Law is a felony subject to both criminal and civil penalties, including exclusion from participation in the Medicare and the Medicaid programs. The federal law also prohibits any payment to a physician as an inducement to limit or reduce necessary medical services to Medicare and Medicaid beneficiaries.

Certain activities have been exempted from the anti-kickback prohibition by either statutory exceptions or "safe harbor" regulations promulgated by HHS OIG.[5] For example, certain personal service contracts or bona fide employment arrangements between hospitals and physicians and the waiver of coinsurance and deductibles, which meet certain criteria, will be safe from enforcement activity. On the other hand, the OIG has issued various Special Fraud Alerts to identify practices that potentially violate the law and to encourage the reporting of suspect activity by means of a toll-free "hot-line" telephone number. For example, a Special Fraud Alert, issued in 1992, lists various types of hospital incentives to physicians that potentially violate the law, including use of free or discounted office space or equipment; provision of free or discounted billing, administrative, or nursing services; certain income guarantees; payment of a physician's travel and expenses for continuing education and conferences; and payment for services, such as administrative or consultative services, that require minimal substantive duties or for which compensation paid exceeds the value of the services. Activity that violates the Anti-Kickback Law may also involve liability under the federal Civil False Claims Act,[6] which prohibits the knowing presentation of a false or fraudulent claim for payment by the government. Violation of the Civil False Claims Act is subject to both criminal and civil penalties.

Federal Self-Referral Prohibition Laws

The federal self-referral prohibition laws[7] are commonly known as the "Stark" laws in recognition of their primary sponsor, Representative Fortney "Pete" Stark (D-Calif.). Stark I, enacted in 1989, prohibits referrals for clinical laboratory services payable under Medicare if the referring physician or an immediate family member of the physician has a financial relationship with the entity performing the services. Stark II, enacted in 1993, extends the prohibition to other designated health services and to services payable under the Medicaid program. The Stark laws are intended to discourage unnecessary utilization of health care services by eliminating financial incentives that may result in such utilization. The Stark laws prohibit the making of a claim for payment of services where there is referral and a financial relationship between the physician and the entity performing the designated health services, irrespective of the intent of the parties to the arrangement.

The designated health services that are subject to the self-referral prohibition include clinical laboratory services; physical therapy services; occupational therapy services; radiology services; radiation therapy services; furnishing of durable medical equipment; parenteral and enteral nutrients, equipment, and supplies; prosthetics, orthotics, and prosthetic devices; home health services; outpatient prescription drugs; and inpatient and outpatient hospital services.

The law defines "referrals" as "the request by a physician for the item or service, including a request for a consultation by a physician," and the "request or establishment of a plan of care" related to any of the designated health services that may be paid by Medicare. Excluded from the definition of referrals are requests by pathologists for clinical laboratory tests and pathological exams, requests by radiologists for diagnostic radiology services, and requests by radiation oncologists for radiation services, where such services are furnished by such pathologist, radiologist, or radiation oncologist. The prohibition is applicable if the referring physician has an ownership or investment interest in or a compensation arrangement with the entity performing the designated health services billed to Medicare or Medicaid.

The Stark laws define a number of exceptions to the self-referral prohibition. There is an exception for referrals for medical services performed or personally supervised by a physician and for referrals for the services of a physician who is a member of the same group practice as the referring physician. There is an exception for ownership interests held in the form of publicly traded securities in entities meeting certain asset requirements. There are exceptions for various types of compensation arrangements, including:

- Certain minor remuneration arrangements (e.g., forgiveness of amounts attributable to inaccurate or mistakenly performed tests or procedures, and provision of supplies or devices used to collect, store, or transport specimens or report test results).

- Rentals of office space and equipment pursuant to a written agreement with a term of at least one year and a rental rate consistent with fair market value.

- Bona fide employment arrangements in which compensation is reasonable and determined without reference to the value or volume of referrals between the parties.

- Personal service arrangements based on a written agreement with a term of at least one year, with compensation set in advance consistent with fair market value and unrelated to the value or volume of referrals by the physician (except as part of a permitted incentive compensation arrangement).

The Stark laws prohibit payment of any claim for services rendered pursuant to a prohibited referral. If such a claim is paid, the amounts collected must be refunded. The law additionally specifies civil monetary penalties for violations. It is anticipated that OIG will promulgate the final regulations to implement Stark II by the year 2000, at which time enforcement of this law may be expected to be a federal priority.

As is evident from the preceding summary, the federal fraud and abuse laws and self-referral prohibition laws are extraordinarily complex, and physicians should obtain legal counsel when contemplating any transaction or arrangement that may be affected by these laws.

Managed Care Contracts

Physicians will encounter myriad managed care arrangements in the evolving health care market. The various entities that may seek to contract with physicians to provide health services to defined groups of persons include traditional third-party payers, such as insurance companies, self-insured companies, third-party administrators, health maintenance organizations, and governmental health programs; and provider networks and "brokers," such as preferred provider organizations, independent practice associations, physician-hospital organizations, integrated delivery systems, and physician practice management companies. The legal, operational, and financial complexities and pitfalls inherent in this array of contractual arrangements should not be underestimated, and it is not prudent for a physician to execute such contracts (and amendments and renewals) without thorough competent analysis that ideally includes consultation with legal and business advisors.

Although the need for caution may seem obvious, physicians will frequently focus only on reimbursement rates and assume that the contract language is standard, innocuous, and nonnegotiable. In addition, physicians may feel they are self-sufficient and have an overpowering aversion to the cost of professional consultation. However, the downside risk and financial consequences to the physician resulting from an improvident, onerous contract can far outweigh an appropriate investment in careful review and negotiation of such arrangements.

Because of the variability and the complexity of managed care contract terms and conditions, this discussion will only generally address the major issues to be considered when evaluating a managed care arrangement. Preliminarily, the physician should assess the managed care organization and the operational implications of the arrangement. The issues to be considered include:

- The organization's financial status (as demonstrated by audited financial statements) and reputation for claims payment.

- Present and projected number of members and expected volume of patient referrals.

- Whether the physician must refer patients within a provider network and, if so, what other physicians and hospitals are in such network.

- Procedures for verification of patient eligibility and identification of who assumes the risk for errors.

- Qualifications of the organization's medical director.

- Utilization review procedures.

- Billing procedures (time frame, format, documentation, and other claims submission requirements).

- Any special requirements relative to appointment availability, office hours, physician and staff qualifications, and record keeping and reporting.

The contract document itself must also be analyzed carefully. The document will typically begin with a paragraph identifying the parties and a preface consisting of a series of recitals or "whereas" clauses describing the parties' respective roles and objectives in the arrangement. An evaluation should be made as to whether all responsible entities are actually included as parties to the contract. Some arrangements may be with brokers and intermediaries and not include the entity that has the financial obligation for the payment of claims.

The contract will normally contain an extensive section providing specific definitions of key words and phrases used in the document. These definitions have a significant bearing on the physician's rights and responsibilities under the arrangement. For example, attention must be given to ensure that the definition of the "covered services" to be provided by the physician is consistent with his or her expectations and capabilities. The definition of "medically necessary" may confer on the managed care organization the authority to retrospectively review services and deny payment based on a unilateral determination that the services were not necessary.

Managed care contracts frequently make reference to and incorporate numerous appendices, exhibits, and other documents. These materials may include a schedule of reimbursement rates, claims submission procedures, utilization review policies, patient grievance procedures, and other managed care organization policies and procedures that are binding on the physician. It is important to ensure that all such materials are received and reviewed.

Other contractual issues that should be considered include:

- Whether the payer has an obligation and an incentive to make payment within a specified, reasonable time following the physician's submission of a "clean" (i.e., proper and complete) claim.

- Whether the contract grants the managed care organization the right to unilaterally change the fee schedule and policies and procedures applicable to the physician and, if so, whether the physician is assured sufficient advance notice of such changes and the option to exit the arrangement if a change is objectionable.

- Whether the contract contains a "Most Favored Nation" clause that obligates the physician to give the managed care organization pricing that is no higher than that provided to any other payer with which the physician contracts.

- Whether the contract allows the managed care organization to offset payments to the physician to adjust for "erroneous" previous payments, such as for retrospective determinations of lack of eligibility or medical necessity, notwithstanding that the physician disputes such action.

- Whether the contract requires the use of internal grievance procedures or arbitration to resolve disputes, including payment issues.

- Whether the contract contains provisions obligating the physician to continue to care for patients following termination of the contract.

Physician's Relationship with Other Providers

Hospital Medical Staff

The organized medical staff is an essential part of the hospital and is required by JCAHO accreditation standards, Medicare and Medicaid Conditions of Participation, and state hospital licensure laws. The medical staff has delegated responsibility for the quality of the professional services provided by individuals with clinical privileges and is accountable to the hospital's governing body, which retains legal responsibility for the quality of patient care in the hospital. A primary function of the medical staff is to establish and participate in the credentialing process for appointment of physicians to the medical staff and in the granting, renewal, and revision of clinical privileges. In particular, the medical staff is generally delegated responsibility to develop the criteria and the review process, subject to governing body approval, and to gather and evaluate information on applicants and members and provide recommendations to the governing body, which has ultimate responsibility to decide the appointment, reappointment, and clinical privileges of members of the medical staff.

A physician is not entitled to practice in a hospital simply because he or she holds a license to practice medicine; he or she must be approved and appointed through the hospital's credentialing process. This process usually consists of the following stages:

- Pre-application, at which time the physician is informed of the hospital's criteria, requirements, and application process.

- Formal application, requiring the physician applicant's submission of extensive data relevant to his or her personal character, education, training, experience, professional competence, and financial responsibility.

- Verification and investigation, at which time the hospital contacts various entities, such as educational institutions, employers, professional peers, other hospitals, malpractice insurance carriers, licensure agencies, and the National Practitioner Data Bank, to confirm and obtain information about the physician applicant.

- Review and recommendation by appropriate medical staff committees, at which time the physician applicant may be requested to meet with the committee to clarify information.

- Action by the governing body. It is critical for the physician applicant to be thorough, forthright, cooperative, and compliant with all mandatory timelines in the credentialing process. The hospital's medical staff bylaws or other policies generally will grant the physician applicant the right to a hearing to challenge an unfavorable recommendation or decision on his or her application.

The hospital's governing board is responsible for determining the hospital's needs for physicians and for establishing policies and plans (based on factors such as the hospital's mission, priorities, and resources and the needs of the community) that may designate specialties or departments as "open" or "closed" to the addition of physicians or limited to physicians who have certain skills or an employment or exclusive contract relationship with the hospital. In addition, the hospital's criteria may include consideration of the physician's use of resources and cost-effectiveness compared to his peers (referred to as "economic credentialing") and other legitimate factors related to the hospital's needs and quality of care.

While the courts are reluctant to intervene relative to hospitals' medical staff decisions, such decisions can be challenged under the antitrust laws. In order to protect the credentialing process against claims that a medical staff decision involves an anti-competitive conspiracy by other physicians, hospitals will ensure that their criteria are appropriate and fairly applied and that the governing board makes the final decision. The federal Health Care Quality Improvement Act of 1986[8] provides immunity from damages under state or federal law—including antitrust, tort, and contract actions, but excluding civil rights actions and government enforcement actions—for various persons and entities involved in professional review activity, which includes actions relative to a physicians' medical staff membership and clinical privileges, provided that certain procedural and substantive standards are met. Many states' laws similarly confer conditional immunity from civil liability to participants in peer review activities.

National Practitioner Data Bank

The National Practitioner Data Bank (NPDB), established by HHS under the Health Care Quality Improvement Act of 1986, is a permanent registry of information required to be reported by health care providers, state licensure agencies, and insurance companies relative to professional malpractice and misconduct by physicians and other health care practitioners. The act requires the following matters to be reported to the NPDB:

- Actions by a state licensure agency to revoke, suspend, or restrict a physician's license for reasons involving the professional competence or conduct of the physician.

- A professional review action by a peer review body that adversely affects a physician's clinical privileges for longer than a 30-day period.

- A physician's surrender of clinical privileges while under investigation.

- Payment by a physician or on behalf of a physician under a policy of insurance or self-insurance, or other settlement or partial settlement in connection with a medical malpractice case.

Hospitals are required to make inquiry to the NPDB for information on physicians and other practitioners at the time of application for medical staff membership or clinical privileges, and at least every two years for current medical staff members. Information contained in the NPDB is generally confidential. Access is granted only to hospitals for practitioners who are applying for or have clinical privileges, to a practitioner for information on himself, to state boards of medical examiners, to health care entities that have or may be entering employment or affiliation relationships with practitioners, and to malpractice litigants under certain conditions.

Antitrust Laws

Of the federal antitrust laws, the Sherman Act[9] and the Federal Trade Commission Act[10] are particularly relevant to physicians. Section 1 of the Sherman Act prohibits contracts, combinations, and conspiracies in restraint of trade. Thus, Section 1 is violated by an agreement or concerted action by two or more individuals or entities to create an unreasonable restraint on trade. Section 2 of the Sherman Act prohibits monopolization and efforts to monopolize by exclusionary or predatory means. The Sherman Act is enforced by the Department of Justice through civil or criminal actions in federal court and may also be enforced by civil actions brought by state attorneys general and private parties. The Federal Trade Commission Act prohibits unfair methods of competition and unfair or deceptive acts or practices. This act is enforced by the FTC through administrative and judicial proceedings. It is a per se violation of the Sherman Act for two or more physicians to engage in price fixing or group boycotts. For example, the U.S. Supreme Court has held that a maximum fee schedule set by agreement of independent physicians in an Arizona medical society was unlawful price fixing.[11]

The formation of joint ventures by physicians and physician groups can raise questions under the antitrust laws. For example, the formation of physician "networks" to market services to health insurance plans could involve agreements on fee schedules in violation of Section 1 of the Sherman Act. It could violate Section 2 of the Sherman Act if a sufficient number of physicians are involved in a monopolization effort. The Department of Justice and the FTC have issued joint policy statements that define certain safe harbors for physician joint ventures.

While employees engaged in collective bargaining with employers are exempt from the antitrust laws, this exemption does not apply to "unions" of independent physicians desiring to collectively negotiate with purchasers of health care. However, there is a rising interest in "unionization" among physicians to cope with the pressures of managed care, and there is some effort to seek an antitrust exemption for such physician unions.

Another area of antitrust issues involves hospital medical staff privileges and peer review. A physician whose staff privileges have been denied, terminated, or reduced may claim that this is due to a conspiracy in restraint of trade, violating Section 1 of the Sherman Act.

Emergency Medical Treatment and Active Labor Act (EMTALA)

As a consequence of the perceived problem of "patient dumping," i.e., hospitals' refusing treatment to medically indigent patients and/or transferring such patients to other charity hospitals, Congress enacted EMTALA[12] in 1985. EMTALA requires hospitals that participate in the Medicare program and that provide emergency services to:

- Screen any person seeking treatment to determine if the person has an emergency medical condition or is in active labor.

- If it is determined that an emergency medical condition exists, to provide the treatment necessary to stabilize the patient or, under certain defined circumstances, provide an appropriate transfer to another health care facility.

These obligations apply to the hospital and to all physicians affiliated with the hospital; however, they do not apply to physician's offices. EMTALA defines the following circumstances under which physicians may face liability:

- Negligent acts by the physician in violation of an EMTALA requirement.

- False certification that the benefits of a transfer outweigh the risks.

- Misrepresentation of a person's condition or other information.

- Failure of an on-call physician to appear within a reasonable time after notification that assistance is needed to address an emergency medical condition.

EMTALA prohibits hospitals from penalizing physicians who refuse to transfer a person with an unstabilized emergency medical condition. While there is no private right of action for civil damages against physicians for violations of EMTALA, physicians are subject to civil monetary penalties and to exclusion from Medicare and state health care programs.

References

1. U.S.C. 1001, *et seq.*

2. *Cruzan v. Director of Missouri Department of Health*, 497 U.S. 261 (1990).

3. 42 U.S.C. 1395 cc.

4. 42 U.S.C. 1320 a-7b, *et seq.*

5. 42 C.F.R. 1001.952

6. 31 U.S.C. 3729, *et seq.*

7. 42 VS.C 1395, *et seq.*

8. 42 U.S.C. 11101, *et seq.*

9. 15 U.S.C. 1 and 2.

10. 15 U.S.C. 45

11. *Arizona v. Maricopa County Medical Socie*ty, 457 V.S. 332 (1982).

12. 42 U.S.C. 1395cc and 1395dd.

Bryan Burgess, JD, MPH, is Executive Advisor, University of South Florida Physicians Group, Tampa, Florida.

Major Trends and Forecasts

Some of the major trends that will drive any forecasts of the health care system are:

- Cost of health care.

- Current status, growth, and future changes in managed care.

- Provider responses to this environment, especially hospitals and physicians.

- Responses of employers, who currently pay some 35 percent of the bill for health care.

- Responses of government, which pays some 45 percent of the price tag, both at the state and federal level.

- Consumer responses to this changing health care environment.

Before jumping into these specific trends, let's review how we got to where we are today.

In the past decade or so, there have been some massive and pervasive changes in how health care is financed, organized, and delivered.

Health Care Delivery in the '70s

Providers—that is, physicians and hospitals—were economically and politically dominant in the health care system (figure 1, page 120). The patient was insured through either an employer or a government program, which paid premiums to an insurance company, which then paid in a fee-for-service arrangement to both physicians and hospitals. The third-party carrier was a very passive entity. When fees from providers went up, they were passed on as increased premiums to employers and the government. There was continuous cost inflation from which the patient was essentially insulated, because these costs were picked up by either government or employers. This scheme fueled the increase in volume and intensity of health services and stimulated medical price growth significantly. Parenthetically, at that time, both patients and physicians were very satisfied and believed that the United States had the best health care available in the world.

Cost versus Access

Since the early 1980s, the United States has faced the issue of rising health care costs without any evidence of increasing access to health care. In fact, there is now growing

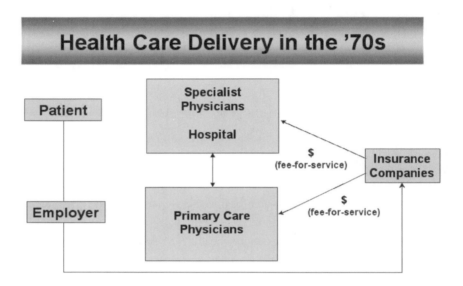

Figure 1

evidence of decreasing access to health care, with somewhere in excess of 16 percent of the population currently uninsured.

This has led to a focus by the payers of this health insurance, largely government and employers, on these costs. Close to 25 percent of all employer benefits are expended on medical benefits. This benefit cost is, of course, embedded in the price of products. When health care costs began to rise in late 1987, peaking in the mid-1990s, it created a significant gap between global sales prices and medical costs. This was a competitive disadvantage for American products in the international market from the employers' perspective.

The federal government was concerned with the same issues. Until recently, the federal government was dealing with a significant deficit and laboring under constant forecasting of the threatened bankruptcy of Medicare.

Medicare Part A Trust Fund

The Medicare trust fund has been projected to be bankrupt in the year 2001. As a consequence of the Balanced Budget Amendments of 1997, it is now projected that the bankruptcy will be delayed to the year 2008-2010.

The states were also seeing more and more of their budgets being consumed by Medicaid, leaving fewer and fewer dollars for other public services.

The Force behind Managed Care

These concerns, driven by supply side economics and fee-for-service medicine, combined with autonomy of providers and patients, drove up the costs of health care at double-digit rates, so that it was projected that health care would consume some 15 percent of the Gross Domestic Product, or approximately $1 trillion dollars annually, before the end of the decade. This created great concern among the two major payers: employers and government.

These forces led to the shift from the supply side, where doctors and hospitals were dominant, to the demand side of the equation, where payers, employers, government, and insurers reside. This shift, with managed care a major driver, was facilitated and made possible by excess capacity on the supply side.

The Doctor Boom

There is a serious excess of physicians in the U.S. civilian population. The number of doctors has risen from some 200,000 in the early 1950s to 400,000+ in 1980s. The number is projected to rise to 730,000 by the year 2000 and to continue to grow. Most important, however, we have gone from some 140 to 150 physicians per 100,000 population to 260+ physicians per 100,000 population, which most believe is a serious physician glut.

The second shift is political. At both the state and national political level, the electorate and politicians are disenchanted with government regulation. It is deemed expensive and inefficient. Under the current political paradigm, one expects market forces to solve all types of problems in the economy as well as societal problems, including health care. In the recent elections and in current debates in both state legislatures and Congress, there does not seem to be any sign of change in how to implement national policy through market forces and privatization. This shift to market forces has been emphasized over and over by Allan Greenspan, Chairman of the Federal Reserve Board, as one of the major reasons for the United States' current booming economy.

Health Care Delivery in the '80s and Early '90s

As a consequence of these forces and issues, health care was reformatted in the late 1980s and early 1990s (figure 2, page 122). This reorganization of financing and delivery of health care is generically called "managed care." The focus of health care

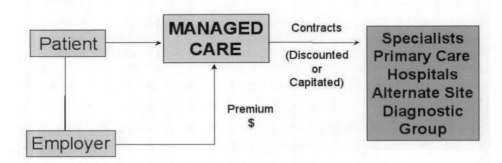

Figure 2

delivery is with managed care companies now acting as intermediaries between patients, employers, and providers of health care. Managed care companies are no longer passive insurers; they manage care through prices by negotiating and brokering contracts with a variety of providers.

It's not likely that there will be a return to the old fee-for-service medicine. Today's physicians will have to learn how to manage and deal with the current competitive, price-driven, managed care market that has replaced it.

There is growing evidence that the unregulated health care market will not be able to keep costs down much longer and that our medical care system will again become expensive and perhaps more inequitable and dysfunctional (figure 3, page 123).

Costs

Under the old supply side economics, it was projected that we would soon spend some 15 percent of the Gross Domestic Product on health care, or in excess of $1 trillion dollars. Here's what really seems to have happened.

In 1996, for the first time, U.S. health care spending did top $1 trillion dollars. However, the percentage increase has ameliorated from the early 1990s, where spending increased almost 9 percent per year, to less than 5 percent per year in 1996. It is believed that health care expenditures have been controlled primarily by a combination of the growth of managed care and the low general inflation rate of all commodities.

If Allan Greenspan and the Federal Reserve Board are correct and their projections hold, total expenditures are projected to go from slightly more than $1 trillion dollars to almost $1.3 trillion dollars, but the growth rate will remain relatively low, between 4 ½ and 5 ½ percent. As a result, health care expenditures will end up somewhere around 13 ½ percent of the Gross Domestic Product (figure 4, page 124).

What's Happened to Indemnity?

Employers, recognizing the potential of managed care to control this fringe benefit cost, have shifted significantly into managed care (figure 5, page 124). As recently as 1992, indemnity made up some 50 percent of health care benefits. However, the percentage decreased to 32 percent in 1994 and was 15 to 18 percent in 1996, with the remaining 80+ percent of the benefit package offered through some sort of managed care mechanism. Currently, there are more than 80 million Americans enrolled in some sort of managed care plan.

A significant percentage of managed care plans are now in financial difficulty (figure 6, page 125). As many as one-half of the nation's 650 HMOs were predicted to lose money in 1998. HMO profit margins, on the average, dipped into the red in 1997.

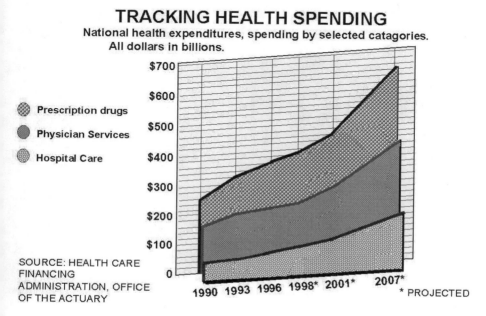

TRACKING HEALTH SPENDING
National health expenditures, spending by selected catagories.
All dollars in billions.

- Prescription drugs
- Physician Services
- Hospital Care

SOURCE: HEALTH CARE FINANCING ADMINISTRATION, OFFICE OF THE ACTUARY

1990 1993 1996 1998* 2001* 2007*

* PROJECTED

Figure 3

National Health Expenditure (NHE) Forecasts, 1996 to 2000

Year	1997 Estimates (dollars in billions)	Growth Rate	NHE as a percentage of GDP[1]
1996	$1,035.1	4.4%	13.6%
1997	1,096.4	5.9	13.6
1998	1,153.1	5.2	13.5
1999	1,221.3	5.9	13.5
2000	1,289.3	5.6	13.5

[1] Assumes real gross domestic product growth of 3% in 1998, 1999 and 2000. GDP is the total value of goods and services produced in the United States.

NOTE: These results are not stated on a per capita basis.

SOURCE: Cookson and Reilly, Milliman & Robertson, March, 1998

Figure 4

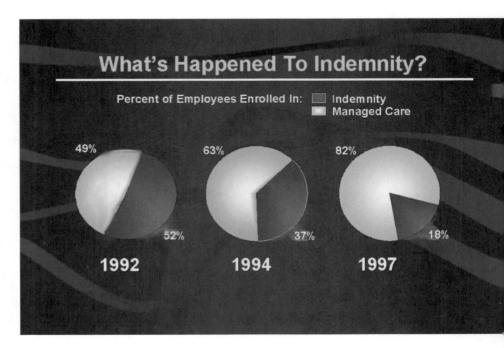

Figure 5

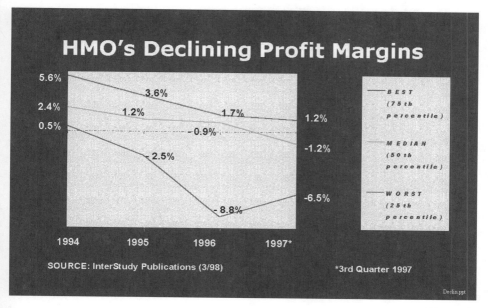

Figure 6

HMOs will try to recoup losses by:

- Imposing premium increases at a level of 4-6 percent or higher, as well as continuing to squeeze down payments to providers. A major example of this is Kaiser Permanente in California, which successfully demanded a double-digit premium increase from California Public Employee Retirement System, the major state employment system benefit package.

- Continue to squeeze hospital and physician payments.

It is projected that, although costs will continue to rise, increases will be moderated and ameliorated by managed care's repositioning itself, as well as by the continued strength of the general economy. As noted, managed care continues to grow and thrive in the private sector, despite its current financial difficulty. Managed care plans, on average, are some 18 percent cheaper than traditional indemnity plans. However, where there has been significant penetration of managed care, such as in Los Angeles and Miami, they are 90+ percent cheaper than indemnity. In the Tampa/St. Petersburg, FL, area, they are some 37 percent cheaper than indemnity. This fact has not escaped the attention of both state and federal governments, which have been enduring 9-10 percent annual increases in costs in their health care programs.

Medicaid Managed Care Growth

Since 1992, Medicaid enrollment has grown to in excess of 30 million people, with almost 15 million people (50 percent of the eligible Medicaid population) enrolled in managed care programs. In the not-to-distant future, that percentage should reach 80-90 percent.

Medicare Managed Care Growth

The federal government has not been far behind in pushing Medicare risk contracts. In 1997, of the nearly 40 million eligible beneficiaries, only 5 million were enrolled in Medicare managed plans. But this is projected to increase to more than 15 million by the year 2007. Many believe this is a conservative estimate as a consequence of the Balanced Budget Amendments of 1997. If that projection is correct, approximately one-third of Medicare eligibles will be in managed care (figure 7, below).

With significant growth in managed care, there has been a significant parallel growth in managed care organizations. Very important, however, much of that growth in the past five years has occurred in the for-profit sector, so that, today, for-profit managed care plans now make up well over 50 percent of all managed care programs. In addition, it is projected that for-profit managed care plans will soon make up some 75 percent of all plans.

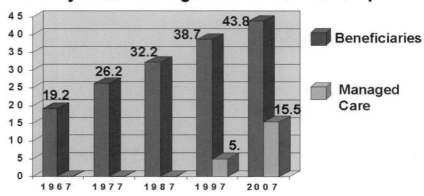

Medicare Population (1967-2007) and Projected Managed Care Membership

Source: Health Care Financing Administration, Office of the Actuary, December 1996

4-29-98.ppt

Figure 7

This shift to the for-profit sector is and should be of great concern, because inherent in any for-profit venture is a requirement of a return on investment, and this return on investment must come from patient care services, the so-called "medical loss ratio." Wall Street profits and the medical loss ratio are major motivating forces and, consequently, a significant concern in the health care marketplace.

This conflict between for-profit and not-for-profit managed care plans is significant, because, in general, not-for-profit managed care plans are ranked higher by enrollees than the for-profit plans in most satisfaction surveys. And not-for-profit plans' medical loss ratios are generally in the range of 90 percent, whereas the for-profits are in the range of 80 percent or lower.

Despite well-publicized media reports of consumer backlash against managed care, most surveys do not demonstrate excessive dissatisfaction of patients with managed care, nor is there any evidence of diminished quality of care in managed care plans. Therefore, the jury is still out on whether the American public is ready to get rid of managed care as the primary health care vehicle or whether the controlled medical loss ratio has, or will have, an adverse impact on health care quality.

Evolution of Managed Care Strategy

There has been a gradual evolution of the strategy of managed care in the marketplace (figure 8, below). In the beginning, managed care was primarily managing costs, as it is

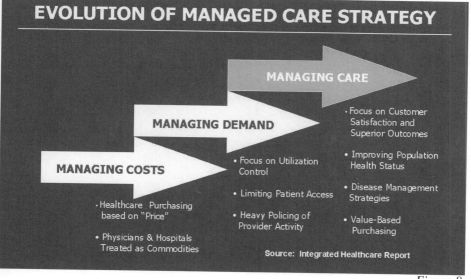

Figure 8

still doing in some markets, with health care purchasing by employers based almost exclusively on price and physicians and with hospitals being treated as commodities. Managed care began focusing on managing demand through utilization and patient access. However, it is predicted that, in the near term, we'll be moving on to managing care—that is, focusing on patient/consumer satisfaction, outcomes from both a medical perspective and a social perspective, and improvements in the health care status of populations. This means getting into disease management and beginning to evaluate products in a value-based purchasing arrangement.

It is predicted that managed care organizations will return to profitability. They will continue to grow in both the public and the private sector. Managed care plans will offer more and more choice to consumers, including decreased use of the gatekeeper strategy, and will respond to general consumer concerns, both through voluntary efforts of managed care plans and probably as a consequence of both state and federal patient protection legislation.

Managed Care Consolidation

Over the past few years, there has been significant consolidation, especially in the for-profit managed care sector. For example, United Healthcare purchased Health Partners of Arizona. Aetna acquired U.S. Healthcare and NYL Care. United Healthcare attempted to acquire Humana, which would have created the largest managed care company in the country. For a variety of reasons, not the least of which was a concern by a variety of state insurance commissioners relative to restraint of trade, the deal did not come to fruition.

On the horizon is the potential purchase by Aetna U.S. Healthcare of Prudential Insurance Company of American for approximately $1 billion. If this deal goes through, the resulting company would be the largest health benefit provider in the nation. Many predict this merger will also be challenged by state and federal agencies. However, in order to move toward profitability, the managed care industry will continue to attempt consolidation as a means of increasing local market dominance and to be able to better control premium pricing and compensation to providers.

Thinning the Ranks of U.S. Hospitals

Since 1987, there has been a significant and progressive number of hospital closures (figure 9, page 131). In addition, there has been a major increase in the number of vertically integrated systems. From 1994 to 1996, there was a 122 percent increase in the number of vertically integrated systems. These systems are primarily aggregates of hospitals. Hotbeds of such aggregation, of course, have been teaching hospitals in Boston, where Beth-Israel and Deaconess system merged, where Massachusetts General

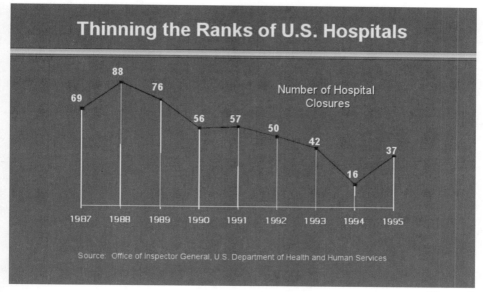

Figure 9

Hospital and Brigham and Women's Hospital merged, etc. Similar activity has occurred in Philadelphia and St. Louis among the academic health centers.

To date, however, the vast majority of these aggregations have not demonstrated evidence of any economies of scale; for the most part have not closed or consolidated redundant and duplicative services; and, in some markets, have not even been able to demonstrate negotiating strength in the market.

To date, large integrated systems' operating margins have been significantly lower than individual U.S. hospital average operating margins. They have not even been able to demonstrate cost savings. Nonetheless, the trend of merger mania, consolidation, and formation of both horizontal and vertically integrated systems persists, with no evidence of decreasing momentum. However, a number of think tanks, health economists, and the public are beginning to doubt and challenge this strategy of integrated systems.

Consumers' Perceptions of Hospital Care

It all comes down to what patients think of hospitals and whether they are getting the service that they want. Patients are intrigued with the technology that's available in hospitals and are impressed with the superb, high-quality doctors, nurses, and other health care professionals that they house. However, and it is a BIG however, they recognize that the health care provided in hospitals is not consistent. They are displeased that hospital staffs act cold, callous, and aloof and that, when they're in the hospital, they had better be their own watchdogs.

In order to make health care more consumer friendly, health care professionals and administrators are trying to follow the example of other industries. Parallels between the health care system and the banking industry are quite striking.

Niche Banking

Major banking consolidations are occurring throughout the United States. At the same time, there is significant growth in niche competition in banking that divide the bank into activities such as asset management, discount brokerage, consumer finance, auto finance, credit cards, mutual funds, separate mortgage services, full service brokerage, capital market management, etc. Just as a bank can be divided into these focused niches that are consumer friendly and easy to access, perhaps the large hospital and the hospital system should follow suit.

Focused Clinical Centers

How can you break the hospital into focused clinical centers? If you believe there is needless proliferation of technology, develop a focused clinical center that uses only necessary and appropriate technology. If you feel, as a patient, that there is very little choice in a large multispecialty tertiary care hospital, you would have a choice of many focused clinical centers. It would be easier to measure quality and costs in a focused clinical center. And fewer legislative and regulatory mandates would be needed, because the focused clinical center would offer considerable choice (figure 10, page 131).

How could traditional integrated complex hospital systems be divided into focused clinical centers (figure 11, page 129)? Population care clinics offer alternative medicine, mid-life women's centers, and senior centers. Specialty diagnostic centers, such as breast diagnostic centers and digestive disorders clinics, could be promoted by "acute moment" marketing. When patients notice chest pain or a breast lump, they would know where to go because of focused marketing of a particular service, not just the services of a large multispecialty system.

Medical centers of excellence, such as for diabetes, congestive heart failure, and cancer, could be developed. Emergency care approaches could include stoke centers or cardiac crisis centers, which are already developing and proliferating. There are also focused surgical centers, which would be based in a simple basic procedure hospital.

Other services that could be put together in this focused manner include alternative medicine, mid-life women's center, senior center, breast diagnostic center, GI disorder

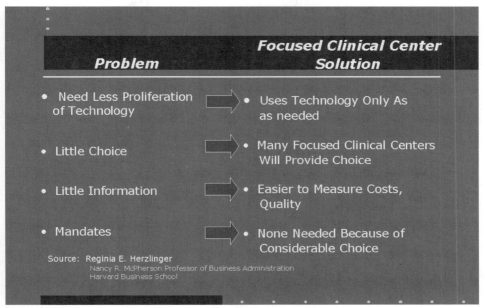

Figure 10

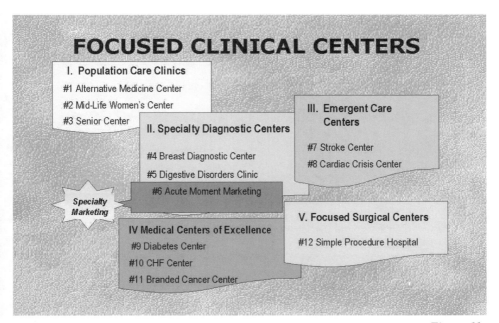

Figure 11

clinic, stroke center, cardiac crisis center, diabetes center, congestive heart failure center, cancer center, and simple procedure hospital. It might even be possible to franchise a clinical service.

Simple Procedure Hospitals

One of the most successful examples of a simple procedure hospital is the HealthSouth Surgical Centers (figure 12, below). Under one roof are operating rooms, inpatient beds, and a rehabilitation center; HealthSouth has contracts with an imaging center in-house. The vast majority of procedures performed are orthopedic. Through this approach, HealthSouth Corporation has become the nation's largest provider of rehabilitative services and has recently increased its outpatient surgical centers by 20 percent by acquiring 34 centers from Columbia/HCA. As a consequence, by the end of 1998, HealthSouth was operating 212 surgical centers in 33 states.

Diabetes Focused Clinical Center

Another example would be a diabetes clinical focus center (figure 13, page 133). This features a multidisciplinary team of endocrinology, renal, cardiovascular, ophthalmology, and other specialists working in multiple sites in the community; in doctors' offices; and, infrequently, in hospitals to treat diabetes in a multidisciplinary, patient-friendly, and focused manner.

Simple Procedure Hospital

HealthSouth Surgical Center of Austin

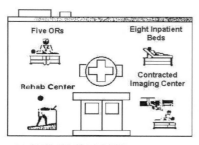

Procedures Performed

✓ ACL repair	>100
✓ Lumbar laminectomy	>80
✓ Cervical laminectomy	>80
✓ Total Knee replacement	>10
✓ Total Hip Replacement	1

- **Opened May 1995**
- **Licensed and reimbursed as acute care hospital**
- **Minority stake held by local specialists**
- **More than 170 inpatient days in first year**

SOURCE: Health Care Advisory Board interviews

Figure 12

Another example of a focused clinical center is in cardiovascular surgery. Many managed care companies and other payers want these types of carve-outs within their managed care plans, because "such arrangements make sense when payers consider that no one tertiary care center does anything well," according to Bradford Koles, Managing Director of The Advisory Board. In a February 1998 report from the Advisory, he goes on to say, "It is odd that we, in health care, thought we should be building conglomerates when the rest of American business is specializing."

Cardiology is a field at the forefront of this focused clinical center trend, because it has complex, but standardized, procedures that lend themselves to a streamlined specific organization. Also, cardiology and cardiovascular surgeries are the fastest growing components of health care costs, exceeding $80 billion dollars per year in expenditures.

Do they work? Well, here's one example: In Dr. Cooley's CABG surgery center, a CABG costs slightly more than $27,000. When performed in a general community hospital, it can cost in excess of $43,000. This is why focused care centers are so attractive.

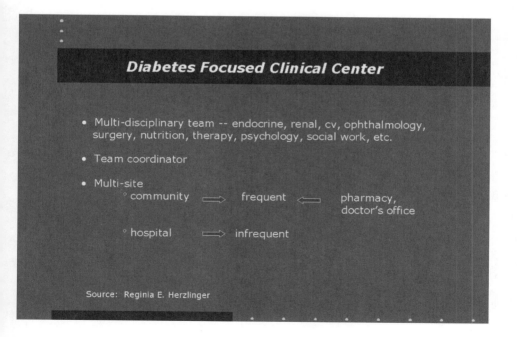

Figure 13

There is a growing consensus that the highly integrated, complex tertiary care system will undergo significant change in the near future and that focused clinical centers will emerge. From a consumer's perspective, from a payer's perspective, and from an employer's perspective, the focused clinical center improves quality and has great potential to reduce costs.

Physician Response

Most Markets Are in Transition

Managed care has moved from low, to medium, to high impact. It begins at the point of low penetration, when there are still busy doctors in fee-for-service arrangements. Indemnity still prevails, but it is becoming more and more limited to geographic areas such as North Dakota and Alaska.

Most markets are in the medium penetration area, where the handwriting is on the wall. Doctors are beginning to get organized into PHOs and IPAs, and alliances are forming. Health care leaders and their organizations are learning how to reposition themselves.

In the high managed care penetration markets, risk arrangements are becoming the vogue, physicians are being deselected as providers, and narrow panels are developing with some direct access to specialists.

As a consequence, solo practice and total physician autonomy are very rapidly disappearing from the American health care scene. New physicians rarely consider starting independent practices. Rather, there has been a very, very steep incline in the growth of physicians aggregating into groups. The number has risen from just over 10 percent in 1965 to 35 percent in 1995.

Physician Group Practice Acquisitions

In addition, physicians are selling their practices. In 1994, there were only 6,000 acquisitions. However, in 1997, almost 28,000 physician practices were sold. Looking at the same period in another way, the number of deals that were done is significant and the number of groups involved well over 500 and growing.

Physician Practices Owned and Managed by Hospitals

The major purchaser of physician practices has been hospitals. Between 1993 and 1995, there was a 172 percent increase in the purchase of physician practices by hospitals, an activity that continues to grow.

After hospitals purchase physician practices, the practices don't seem to have much of an operating margin. However, when physician management companies, such as PhyCor, purchase physician practices, they do have a positive, although somewhat modest, margin of profit (figure 14, below).

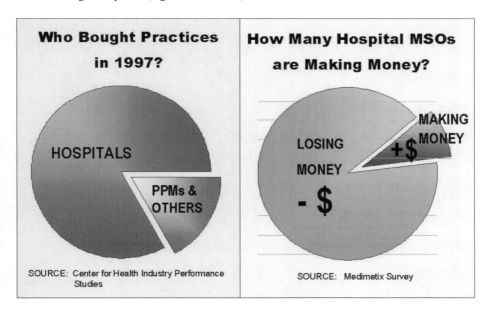

Figure 14

How are these purchases doing? Very poorly. Well over 80 percent of hospitals that have purchased physician practices are losing money, in the range of $50,000 to $100,000 per practice per year. Nonetheless, the trend continues.

The 1997 distribution of physicians by type of practice and employer breaks down as follows (figure 15, page 136):

• Approximately 26 percent of physicians remain in solo practice.

• Approximately 31 percent of physicians are in independent group practice.

• Five percent are operating as independent contractors.

• Approximately 38 percent are in some employed relationship with HMOs, hospitals, medical schools, government, etc.

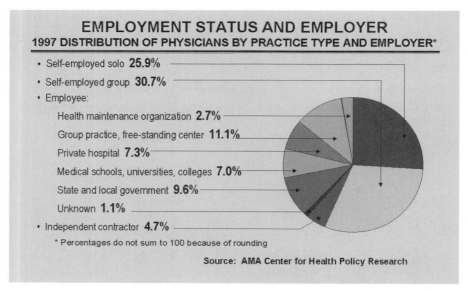

Figure 15

Provider-Sponsored Organizations (PSOs)

Where this will all go, of course, is anybody's guess, and everybody is guessing. One of the guesses is that there will be an emergence, as a result of pressures from business and

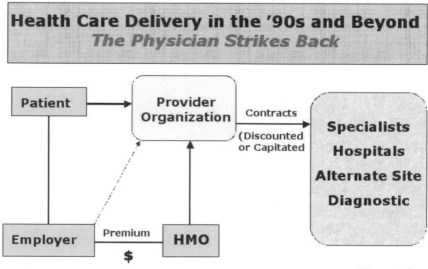

Figure 16

government, especially through Medicare, of provider organizations (figure 16, page 136). The provider organization of the future would consist of physicians and hospitals. The aggregates could be a combination of physician practice management companies, hospitals with employed physicians, or hospitals with PHO relationships. Provider organizations would be the focus and would contract to offer patient services to patients directly, to employers directly, to the federal government directly for Medicare and Medicaid, and to managed care directly. They would subcontract with an entire set of integrated delivery sites, specialists, hospitals, and some of the focused clinical sites I mentioned earlier.

There is no question that provider organizations will be a future configuration that will be tried by many, but they have a very high risk and high reward potential. A sobering insight has been the experience to date. A significant proportion of doctor-owned and doctor-sponsored health care delivery system plans have failed for a number of reasons, but lack of capital for success in a specific market has been a leading cause.

On the other hand, there is a significant amount of physician frustration relative to their loss of autonomy and their obvious loss of power in negotiating in the system. Some will resist forming large groups; selling their practices to physician practice management companies or hospitals; or joining provider-sponsored organization configurations. Rather, they will look toward unionization as a methodology to combat their feeling of hopelessness in the marketplace. This is viewed as a mixed future prediction, because unionization per se and all that it means, such as strikes, have been somewhat antithetical to the medical profession over the years. However, the trend shows growth both nationally and in some specific regions, such as the Northwest. The movement is beginning to grow with some vigor in Florida.

Employers' Response

As mentioned earlier, employers, because they pick up some 35 percent of the health care tab, are major players in influencing trends in and the future of health care. From the employer's point of view, cost is still the most significant factor in selecting health plans. Member services and access run a distant second. Quality measurements are way down on the scale of importance, at least from employers' perspective.

So what are some of the trends and the impact of these trends in employer-sponsored health insurance? The percentage of people with employer health insurance is diminishing. It is projected that the number of employees with employer coverage will be down to some 50 percent by the year 2000. Obviously, with the fall of employer coverage, there will be a proportional increase in the percentage of uninsured persons.

Employers are opting out of funding health insurance because their premium contributions have risen, forcing them to shift premium costs to employees. As a consequence, more than 15 percent of all persons under age 65 are without health insurance, which affects somewhere between 40 and 45 million Americans, most between the ages of 20 and 44, the core of the working group (figure 17, below).

Percentage of Uninsured Americans
July 1996 to July 1997
by Age Group

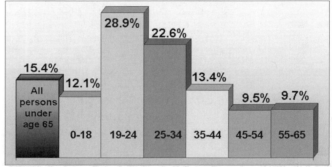

SOURCE: Cunningham, Center for Studying Health System Change, Issue Brief No. 12, April 1998

Figure 17

Some employers are not offering insurance at all; others are outsourcing various work force functions in order not to offer benefits; and many are utilizing increasing numbers of temporary employees, which also decreases the necessity to offer benefit packages.

Another trend is that employers are creating employer coalitions. Currently, there are some 80,000 employers in coalitions that include some 22 million employees. In addition, there is a growing interest in health insurance purchasing cooperatives. More and more states have passed legislation to allow development of health insurance purchasing cooperatives.

One of the most active of these groups is the Buyers Healthcare Action Group (BHCAG) in Minneapolis, which represents 28 major employers in the Twin Cities. These employers, through a variety of mechanisms, have been shifting their employees into less expensive health care insurance programs. For example, 10 BHCAG employers require employees choosing higher cost plans to pay the difference in cost between their choice and lower cost plans. Within cost categories, quality rating was a significant factor. For example, one high-cost system was ranked lower on quality and, as a result, lost 20 percent of its enrollees. The American Medical Association recently suggested moving away from employment-based insurance entirely, a radical and improbable outcome.

Government Response

As noted, government, between the state and the federal levels, picks up approximately 45 percent of the health care tab and has been increasing its outlays in approximately 9-10 percent increments annually. It has not been lost upon government that employers did not see the same kind of increases when they shifted their benefit package to managed care. It is not surprising, therefore, that both state and federal governments have begun to explore, and pursue with vigor, shifting their burdens to a managed care model.

State Government

Medicaid Managed Care Growth

Since 1992, Medicaid enrollment has remained in excess of 30 million individuals (figure 18, below). Medicaid managed care growth has been very rapid and now numbers almost 15 million people, or close to 50 percent of the eligible Medicaid population. The states leading in the move to Medicaid managed care are Tennessee, Arizona, Oregon, Pennsylvania, and Florida, which has begun to shift almost 100 percent of its Medicaid eligibles into some sort of managed care package.

MEDICAID MANAGED CARE GROWTH

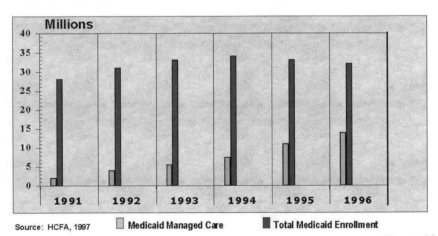

Source: HCFA, 1997 ☐ Medicaid Managed Care ■ Total Medicaid Enrollment

Figure 18

Uninsured Population

Nationally, almost 23 percent of people under 18 are uninsured. All states have been struggling with the problem of "the pediatric" uninsured population. As a consequence of recent legislation, including the Balanced Budget Amendments of 1997, a variety of federal matches to state programs have evolved to address the pediatric uninsured problem. Florida has addressed this coverage gap through a jigsaw puzzle-type approach. The major focus is Medicaid, but also added were Florida Healthy Kids and MediKids to fill in the gaps.

Federal Government

The federal government has been concerned about the future viability of the Medicare program from at least three perspectives:

- The cost of the program has been rising at the rate of 9-10 percent per year, in contrast to the private sector, where increases have ranged from 2-4 percent per year.

- The earlier projection that Medicare bankruptcy would occur by the year 2001. Despite the effects of the Balanced Budget Amendment of 1997, which extended the potential life span of Medicare to 2008-2010, protecting this very significant federal social program is a major priority.

- The knowledge that there will be a significant influx of "baby boomers" into the Medicare-eligible pool, which adds greater pressure on maintaining the viability of this critical program.

It is projected that health, as a percentage of the Gross Domestic Product, will gradually increase from its current level of 13+ percent to close to 15 percent, which is a significantly greater growth than the CPI. As these costs increase, the question will be how they will be handled in the Medicare program.

This increase in health care costs will be compounded by a change in the population mix from the year 2000 on. As the total population grows, most significant is the increasing percentage of the population over 65, which will result in doubling of the number of people eligible for Medicare between 2000 and 2050.

Perhaps even more striking is significant growth in the population 85 years of age and older who will be in the Medicare-eligible pool. That age bracket will create significant demands on the Medicare entitlement package.

Medicare Risk Contract Enrollment Growth

The current trend is the beginning of a significant shift of Medicare enrollees from traditional fee-for-service arrangements to risk/managed care plans. From a modest beginning 10 years ago, there are now approximately 5 million elderly enrolled in Medicare managed care plans. However, by the year 2005, this is expected to increase to more than 15 million Medicare eligibles in managed care plans. This would amount to approximately one-third of potential beneficiaries.

Despite some enrollees' shifting between traditional Medicare and managed care, the general trend in major surveys is that Medicare eligibles are satisfied with the managed care programs, primarily because it gives them extra benefits at less cost.

Included in the Balanced Budget Amendments of 1997 were two major thrusts relative to the future of Medicare. First was the creation of the National Bipartisan Committee on the Future of Medicare. The committee has been convened and is looking not only at how to salvage this important program for the elderly but also at its current structure.

Second, a whole new series of Medicare options were approved in the legislation. Prior to the Balanced Budget Amendment modifications, Medicare consisted of:

- Medicare Part A and Part B, the traditional fee-for-service option.

- Medicare risk managed care contracts, which have been growing.

- Some other minor Medicare programs that have not really caught on.

Why Medicare+Choice?

Congress, recognizing the issues that are evolving relative to Medicare, felt that it should offer some new options and developed a program called Medicare+Choice, now shortened to Medicare C, as opposed to the previous Medicare A and B. The option was proposed:

- To attempt to save money.

- To modernize Medicare so that it is in the mainstream with the other modifications of health care benefits in the United States.

- To offer beneficiaries more choices.

- To create a competitive marketplace for Medicare.

- To expand Medicare managed care into rural areas.

- To respond to political pressure.

- To set the stage for future reform and begin to tinker with a "defined contribution program."

The latter two changes will be referred to the National Bipartisan Committee on Medicare for discussion and recommendations.

In general, what are the new Medicare+Choice general provisions?

- It ends the required 50/50 enrollment split that is currently required for Medicare plans. This means that any Medicare plan must also include enrollment of 50 percent of private sector plans.

- There is going to be a significant switch in the payment rate to end averaging, what Medicare calls average adjusted per capita cost (AAPCC), and to begin to inject risk adjustment.

- It calls for development of quality information that will be available to the consumer.

- It will mount a massive public information campaign, so that those 65 years of age and older will be able to understand what their new options are and can make informed decisions—a major challenge.

- It will have a single, coordinated, annual open enrollment date and will lock in enrollees for the year, after the year 2002.

- It will develop detailed data and risk adjusters.

The entire set of Medicare options that was available beginning January 1, 1999 was:

- The original Medicare A and B.

- The current Medicare health maintenance risk contracts.

- Addition of managed care point of service option.

- Preferred provider organizations.

- Provider-sponsored organizations.

- Private fee-for-service plan.

- Extension of the medical savings account approach.

Original Medicare A and B

Under the first option, beneficiaries can use any physician and any hospital. Physicians and hospitals are paid on a modified fee-for-service basis, but the payment amount is regulated and set by the government.

Health Maintenance Organization Option

Traditional risk contracts are typical HMO approaches in which patients must use doctors and hospitals on the provider list of the HMO, but the plan may pay for prescription drugs and other items not covered by Medicare. This has been one of the major attractions for current Medicare enrollees to shift to the managed care model, because it eliminates the need for MediGap insurance.

HMO with Point of Service Option

This is one of the new Medicaid C options. It is a typical managed care plan, but patients can go outside the network if they're willing to pay extra to see a physician or go to a hospital of their choice that's not on the approved list.

Preferred Provider Organization

This is typical of many private employer programs in which beneficiaries may use any doctors or hospitals but are charged less if they use doctors and hospitals on an approved list. In Medicare C, it's called a Coordinated Care Plan rather than a preferred provider organization.

Provider-Sponsored Organizations or "PSO Option"

A provider-sponosred organization (PSO) is an entity organized by a group of affiliated providers that directly supplies a "substantial proportion" of the benefit package. The providers share the financial risk and must have a majority financial interest in the PSO. The health plan is owned and operated by doctors and hospitals, which supply most of the services to beneficiaries.

Schematically, in the center is the PSO, which is governed by hospitals and physicians. It does direct risk contacting with managed care companies, employers, and government and then contracts for services from physicians and hospitals for diagnostic, ancillary home care, etc. However, it must have insurance-like functions called MSO/ASO functions in order to successfully manage risk.

The real questions are:

- Will PSOs have the capacity to manage risk?

- If they do it well, will they begin to look like, taste like, and smell like the current managed care companies that they are trying to displace? If they find that they are no different in either behavior or character from traditional managed care organizations, what has their creation really achieved?

There was significant lobbying by hospitals and physicians to have this option put into Medicare. As mentioned earlier, employers have also been pushing for this option in order to directly contract with providers and bypass managed care companies. There is great cynicism in the industry as to whether this option, although demanded by the provider side of the equation to put more power back in the supply side as mentioned earlier, will be successful.

There have been many failed attempts by hospitals and physicians to manage insurance risk. In 1997, of 30 provider-sponsored organizations monitored, 40 percent lost money and 20 other hospital-owned provider-sponsored organizations have been losing money. There are many cynics who believe that PSOs provide an excellent opportunity for providers to lose their shirts. Nonetheless, it will be pursued and vigorously promoted by hospital-physician coalitions.

Private Fee-for-Service Plan

Private fee-for-service plans are a major new twist that have received much physician interest. Under these plans, patients may go to any doctor or hospital. The providers themselves are not at risk. However, the beneficiaries would have substantial costs, because there is no control of charges. Therefore, "balanced billing payments" would be requested by providers. The plan gets a fixed amount of federal money for each beneficiary, and physicians and hospitals can charge essentially what they would like and collect the balance from the patient.

Obviously, this may be very attractive for affluent Medicare eligibles, because it is truly the "Cadillac" health plan and a return to the good old days of the physician-patient relationship. Although physicians will applaud this option, it is predicted that market interest will be minimal.

Medical Savings Account

The medical savings account option is already in demonstration around the country, in both the private and the public sectors. Under this option, beneficiaries choose a private insurance policy, which is a high-deductible, catastrophic insurance plan. Medicare pays the premium for the catastrophic coverage and then deposits additional dollars in a medical savings account, which the individual may use to pay routine medical expenses. If, in any given year, the medical savings account is insufficient to meet medical bills, the patient will be responsible for paying the remainder.

Again, this is a proposal that has been pushed forward by market-focused economists. However, to date, not many individuals, either in the public or the private sector, have picked up this option. It is essentially equivalent to an IRA savings approach.

Future of Medicare

What then is the future of Medicare? As mentioned, the National Bipartisan Committee on the Future of Medicare is looking at many options. First of all, it will review and monitor the success of Medicare C. In addition, it will be looking at such things as increasing the Medicare-eligible age from 65 to 67 years. There is great concern, however, that this step will produce a new group of uninsured Americans.

The committee will also examine President Clinton's proposal to allow 55-64-year- olds to buy into the Medicare program under a set of specific conditions. One of the most important options it will be looking at is changing the entire Medicare program from defined benefits to defined contributions (premium support model).

Currently, in both the private sector (employers) and the federal sector, health plans are primarily defined benefits. That is, the employer or the government guarantees a set of benefits to the enrollee. As mentioned earlier, employers, and now the federal government, are very seriously considering moving to a "defined contribution" approach. In a defined contribution approach, the employer and/or government annually commits to a fixed amount for each individual enrollee. The enrollee then has a choice of health plans, some which will be equal to the defined contribution and others of which will have costs greater than the defined contribution. In the latter case, the individual will have to pay out of pocket.

On the federal side of the equation, almost all federal employees are in a defined contribution program called the Federal Employee Health Benefits Plan (FEHBP).

Federal Employee Health Benefits Plan (Premium Support Model)

FEHBP currently covers 2.7 million people and involves some 400 health plans. The government pays up to 75 percent of the cost, and enrollment is available during an annual open enrollment process. Because members of Congress and other federal employees are involved in the FEHBP program and are very pleased with it, they are seriously considering make this THE major thrust of Medicare in the future.

Consumers' Responses and Demand

Last, but far from least, is the current rise in consumerism in the United States. In the medical field, the consumer is the patient. It is now accepted that consumerism is a topic that can no longer be ignored by insurers, providers, or the government. One of the major fuelers of consumerism is baby boomers, who are growing older but have not decreased their demanding style in all facets of the economy; health care is no exception.

What do consumers want? They want convenience. In other words, they want health care to be available when they want it, where they want it, and how they want it. They want information. They want to know what they're getting and why they're getting it, and they want both physical and emotional support. In addition, they want all of this at reduced costs and high quality.

This is quite a set of demands, but most people in industry feel that these consumer desires will have to be met by any successful element of the economy, including the health care sector, be it hospitals, physicians, government, employers, or insurance companies.

Major concerns of Americans lie in ensuring freedom of choice in who provides their health care and in their ability to afford health care without suffering financial hardship. They do believe, however, that quality will increase and that needed treatments will be available when they need them. The public's attitude toward managed care, however, is decidedly mixed.

A headline from *USA Today* is an example: "The New Untouchables—Why You Can't Sue Your HMO." The managed care industry is the only industry in the country that has a congressionally mandated shield from liability. Although, in a recent study of more than 180 health plans in 20 different markets, managed care received better scores than PPOs, fee-for-service arrangements, and point-of-service plans, there will be a push at both the state and the federal levels for patient/consumer protection legislation.

President Clinton appointed an Advisory Commission on Consumer Protection and Quality, which made a series of recommendations called the Consumer Bill of Rights and Responsibilities. Clinton, by Executive Order, has imposed these consumer protections on all federal programs—that is, Medicare, Medicaid, Department of Defense, and VA programs. Clinton, in his January 1998 State of the Union Address, stated, "You have the right to know all of your medical options, not just the cheapest. You have the right to choose the doctor you want for the care you need. You have the right to emergency care, wherever and whenever you need it. And you have the right to keep your medical records confidential."

How the Patient Protection Bills Stack Up

Three major patient protection bills, offered by both Democrats and Republicans, went before the 105th Congress. There seems to be a bipartisan push for some legislation that has continued into the 106th Congress. The big issues are whether these patient protection rights should be imposed on Employee Retirement Income Security Act (ERISA) plans and whether they should preempt state laws. However, there is general agreement to include the prudent lay person provision for emergency care; guaranteed access to specialty care; provisions for external appellate review mechanism; prohibition of gag clauses; and the potential ability to sue managed care plans.

This final issue is important. Some states, such as Texas, have already approved the ability to sue managed care plans, but, if the national legislation passes, it will be available in all states. This issue will be hotly debated in Congress, with employers and insurers stating that it is a bad regulation, the intrusion of government into regulating health care, which should be a market-based commodity, and a source of increased costs.

Consumers, on the other hand, are demanding it and demonstrating that the price tag, at least as currently laid out, seems to be minimal—less than 1 percent per person per year—if the law is enacted as proposed. In addition, consumers are going to become more knowledgeable, some with some good information and some with bad information, a lot of the information coming from the Internet. They will be confronting physicians, hospitals, and other providers with this information and requiring intelligent, "evidence-based" responses.

Disease Management

The new trend toward what is called "disease management" can be seen as a response to consumer demands. The key to disease management is the so-called 80/20 percent rule—20 percent of diseases, primarily chronic diseases, represent 80 percent of the resources expended in health care. If you can address chronic diseases in an organized manner, you have the potential not only to achieve better outcomes but also to lower costs, therefore meeting consumer demands for high quality at reduced costs.

Disease management is a system to coordinate and improve all of the services provided to a patient for a given disease across the entire continuum of care.

Disease management would increase health care value, because it would balance the quality of clinical, economic, service, and humanistic outcomes with the overall costs of those outcomes.

Disease management can be succinctly defined as "a knowledge-based or evidence-based process intended to improve continually the value of health care delivery from the perspective of those who receive it, purchase it, provide it, and evaluate it."

Disease management spans prevention, illness management, and recovery across the spectrum of outpatient, hospital, skilled nursing facility, and home care and coordinates care between the office, the hospital, and other service sites.

The emergence and adoption of disease management shifts to "managing the patient with the disease or diseases" rather than what we currently do, which is "manage a disease in the patient."

The outcomes of care approach of disease management has the already demonstrated potential to improve prognosis and decrease mortality; decrease the use of emergency departments and hospitalization; increase the level of patient functioning; increase adherence to the treatment, whether dietary, drug, or physical activity; increase satisfaction with care; and decrease costs. These elements of disease management have been demonstrated in a number of areas, such as diabetes, asthma, congestive heart failure, and low back pain.

As a consequence, there has been a significant increase in utilization of disease management programs by managed care plans. The major focuses have been on asthma, high-risk pregnancy, diabetes, congestive heart failure, breast cancer, and depression. It is predicted that this trend will continue and expand, because the disease management approach increases quality while decreasing costs for these chronic illnesses under an organized program of care.

Disease management also links with the focused clinical centers noted under the hospital sector of the future. Through disease management, there is a shift of responsibility from primary care physicians as gatekeepers to specialty care access for these chronic diseases. As stated, this trend is being driven by recognition of consumer preference to access a physician of choice—especially a specialist, if they have a known chronic condition.

Disease management addresses consumer disillusionment and anger about the effectiveness of prior authorization and precertification. There are also data to support the belief that, in chronic illnesses, specialists offer higher quality, more cost-effective care than do general primary care physicians.

Consumerism will drive not only other sectors of the economy but also health care. Providers, on the supply side, and insurers, on the demand side, will be required to be more responsive to the demand of consumers for knowledge, choice, quality, and price if they wish to be successful in the new marketplace.

Conclusion

I have tried to outline some of the major trends of today and expand them into some short-term future forecasts. I have focused on the fact that, with the rise of the baby boomers, consumerism will become a major factor. This trend will grow as the population grows and continues to age. Consumers will continue to express concerns about managed care and its rationing and will demand protection. As a consequence, as I noted, consumers will want access and convenience; they will want "express care"; they will want specialty-focused centers; they will want an unconventional hospital, perhaps a medical mall concept; and they will want competition to focus on service as well as on price.

The American public will demand the fixing of Medicare so that its solvency will be ensured for them as they grow older. The debate between for-profit and not-for-profit issues relative to quality and access will continue. As a consequence, "managed competition," the cornerstone of the 1993 Clinton health care reform package, will again be placed on the table for debate as a way of linking the market, choice, and consumer protection.

The government will not lose its concerns about fraud and abuse.. Expansion of the Stark laws will continue, because all are convinced that a significant amount of cost is being consumed through fraudulent activities. Estimates of the cost of these fraudulent activities were in the range of $20 billion in 1997.

The public will continue to be concerned about health care. People are worried about losing insurance coverage. They are confused about what type of health insurance they have or what kind of health insurance they will have, and only one-third of Americans are confident that they will have access to high-quality health care in the next 10 years. And that group is coupled with some 40+ percent of the population who are not confident of their ability to afford health care in the next 10 years without undue hardship.

As a consequence, the American public is increasingly worried about losing health insurance and paying for care if they lack coverage and fretting about the quality of care they will receive, even if they are insured.

Also, constantly lurking in the background is the growing number of uninsured, more than 16 percent of the population, or in excess of 40 million Americans. Many American are concerned that they will soon join that group.

The debate about whether managed care is in or out will continue. Eli Ginzberg eloquently reviewed this situation, and stated his concerns that managed care has not met its promise to the American public.[1] But, in the same journal, an editorial read, "That may be true, but what is the replacement that will achieve quality, cost control, and access?"

Will managed care be replaced by direct contracting and provider- sponsored organizations as being promoted, as mentioned earlier, by the Buyers Healthcare Action

Group in the Twin Cities and the California Public Employees Retirement System. Or will these PSO efforts fail, as predicted by some?

Will there be a massive change in the entire approach to health care in the United States, such as moving away from employment-based insurance by changing the tax code to make providing health insurance a disadvantage, is being suggested by the American Medical Association and others? A similar proposal is being pushed very strongly by Republicans as the only way to address the problem of the 40+ million uninsured, which they believe will continue as long as employment-based insurance is the foundation of private insurance.

Will major reform occur on the premise that health care is a major issue of public interest and that the regulatory model used for the oversight of public utilities should be applied to health care? The argument is that health care merits more regulation than it currently faces because it involves essential services, that interruption of services causes harm, and that the industry receives significant influx of tax revenue.

Yogi Berra once said, "The most difficult thing to predict is the future." It is impossible to know which avenues will be pursued, but most people believe that the pressure of the patient as a consumer will be the major modulating force for the future delivery systems in health care. Conventional wisdom clearly indicates that, if the consumer is not pleased with the product, the enterprise will fail.

Reference

1. Ginzberg, E. "The Uncertain Future of Managed Care." *New England Journal of Medicine* 340(2):144-6, Jan. 14, 1999.

Managed Care Glossary

Administrative Costs
Costs related to utilization review, insurance marketing, medical underwriting, agents' commissions, premium collection, claims processing, insurer profit, quality assurance programs, and risk management.

Adverse Selection
Among applicants for a given group or individual program, the tendency for those with an impaired health status, or those who are prone to higher than average utilization of benefits, to be enrolled in disproportionate numbers in lower deductible plans.

Agency for Health Care Policy and Research (AHCPR)
The agency of the U.S. Public Health Service responsible for enhancing the quality, appropriateness, and effectiveness of health care services.

Ambulatory Care
Health care services provided on an outpatient basis. No overnight hospital stay is required. The services of ambulatory care centers, hospital outpatient departments, physicians' offices, and home health care services fall under this heading.

Beneficiary
Individual who either is using or is eligible to use insurance benefits, including health insurance benefits, under an insurance contract.

Benefit Payment Schedule
List of amounts an insurance plan will pay for covered health care services.

Capitation
A payment system whereby managed care plans pay health care providers a fixed amount to care for a patient over a given period. Providers are not reimbursed for services that exceed the allotted amount. The rate may be fixed for all members, or it can be adjusted for age and gender of the member, based on actuarial projections of medical utilization.

Case Management
The process by which all health-related matters of a case are managed by a physician, a nurse, or a designated health professional. Physician case managers coordinate designated components of health care, such as appropriate referral to consultants, specialists, hospitals, and ancillary providers and services. Case management is intended to ensure continuity of services and accessibility to overcome rigidity,

fragmented services, and misutilization of facilities and resources. It also attempts to match the appropriate intensity of services with the patient's needs over time.

Claims Review
The method by which an enrollee's health care service claims are reviewed prior to reimbursement. The purpose is to validate the medical necessity of the provided services and to be sure the cost of the service is not excessive.

Closed Panel
Medical services are delivered in the HMO-owned health center or satellite clinic by physicians who belong to a specially formed, but legally separate, medical group that only serves the HMO. This term usually refers to a group- or staff-model HMO.

Coinsurance
A cost-sharing requirement under a health insurance policy that provides that the insured will assume a portion or percentage of the costs of covered services. After the deductible is paid, this provision forces the subscriber to pay for a certain percentage of any remaining medical bills, usually 20 percent.

Community Rating
Setting insurance rates based on the average cost of providing health services to all people in a geographic area without adjusting for each individual's medical history or likelihood of using medical services.

Concurrent Review
Review of a procedure or hospital admission done by a health care professional (usually a nurse) other than the one providing the care.

Coordination of Benefits
Provisions and procedures used by third-party payers to determine the amount payable to each payer when a claimant is covered under two or more group health plans.

Copayment
A type of cost-sharing that requires the insured or subscriber to pay a specified flat dollar amount, usually on a per unit of service basis, with the third-party payer reimbursing some portion of remaining charges.

Cost Sharing
The general set of financing arrangements whereby the consumer must pay out-of-pocket to receive care, either at the time of initiating care, during the provision of health care services, or both. Cost sharing can also occur when an insured pays a portion of the monthly premium for health care insurance.

Cost Shifting

Charging one group of patients more in order to make up for underpayment by others. Most commonly, charging some privately insured patients more to make up for underpayment by Medicaid or Medicare.

Credentialing

The process of reviewing a practitioner's credentials, i.e., training, experience, or demonstrated ability, for the purpose of determining if criteria for clinical privileging are met.

Deductible

The out-of-pocket expenses that must be borne by an insurance subscriber before the insurer will begin reimbursing the subscriber for additional expenses.

Diagnosis-Related Groups (DRGs)

A system used by Medicare and other insurers to classify illnesses according to diagnosis and treatment. All Medicare inpatient hospital operating costs are determined in advance and paid on a per-case basis, according to a fixed amount or weight established for each DRG.

Early and Periodic Screening, Diagnosis, and Treatment (EPSDT)

A program that covers screening and diagnostic services to determine physical or mental defects in recipients under age 21, as well as health care and other measures to correct or ameliorate any defects and chronic conditions discovered.

Employee Retirement Income Security Act (ERISA)

ERISA exempts self-insured health plans from state laws governing health insurance, including contribution to risk pools, prohibitions against disease discrimination, and other state health reforms.

Exclusions

Clauses in an insurance contract that deny coverage for select individuals, groups, locations, properties, or risks.

Exclusive Provider Organization (EPO)

A managed care organization that is organized similarly to PPOs, in that physicians do not receive capitated payments, but that only allows patients to choose medical care from network providers. If a patient elects to seek care outside the network, he or she will not be reimbursed for the cost of the treatment.

Exclusivity Clause
Part of a contract that prohibits physicians from contracting with more than one managed care organization.

Experience Rating
A system whereby an insurance company evaluates the risk of an individual or group by looking at the applicant's health history.

Federally Qualified HMOs
HMOs that meet certain federally stipulated provisions aimed at protecting consumers, e.g., providing a broad range of basic health services, assuring financial solvency, and monitoring the quality of care. HMOs must apply to the federal government for qualification. The process is administered by the Health Care Financing Administration (HCFA), Department of Health and Human Services (HHS).

Fee Disclosure
Physicians and caregivers discuss their charges with patients prior to treatment.

Fee for Service
The traditional payment method, whereby patients pay doctors, hospitals, and other providers for services rendered and then bill private insurers or the government.

Fee Schedule
A comprehensive listing of fees used by either a health care plan or the government to reimburse physicians and/or other providers on a fee-for-service basis.

Fiscal Intermediary
The managed care plan that has contracted with providers of service to process claims for reimbursement under health care coverage. In addition to handling financial matters, it may perform other functions, such as providing consultative services or serving as a center for communication with providers and making audits of providers' needs.

Formulary
A list of selected pharmaceuticals and their appropriate dosages deemed to be the most useful and cost effective for patient care. Organizations often develop formularies under the aegis of pharmacy and therapeutics committees. In HMOs, physicians are often required to prescribe from formularies.

Gatekeeper
A primary care physician responsible for overseeing and coordinating all aspects of a patient's medical care. In order for a patient to receive a specialty care referral or hospital admission, the gatekeeper must authorize the visit, unless there is an emergency.

Group Insurance

Any insurance policy or health services contract by which groups (and often their dependents) are covered under a single policy or contract, issued by their employer or another group entity.

Group-Model HMO

An HMO that contracts with a multispecialty medical group to provide care for HMO members; members are required to receive medical care from a physician within the group unless a referral is made outside the network.

Inpatient Services

Inpatient hospital services are items and services furnished to an inpatient of a hospital by the hospital, including bed and board, nursing and related services, diagnostic and therapeutic services, and medical or surgical services.

Health Maintenance Organization (HMO)

An organization that offers prepaid, comprehensive health coverage for both hospital and physician services. An HMO contracts with health care providers (physicians, hospitals, and other health professionals), and members are required to use participating providers for all health services. Members are enrolled for a specific period. Model types include staff, group practice, network, and IPA.

Health Plan Employer Data and Information Set (HEDIS)

A set of performance measures designed to standardize the way health plans report data to employers. HEDIS now measures five major areas of health plan performance: quality, access and patient satisfaction, membership and utilization, finance, and descriptive information on health plan management.

Hold Harmless Clause

A clause frequently found in managed care contracts whereby the HMO and the physician hold each other not liable for malpractice or corporate malfeasance if either of the parties is found to be liable. Many insurance carriers exclude this type of liability from coverage. It may also refer to language that prohibits the provider from billing patients if their managed care companies becomes insolvent. State and federal regulations may require this language.

Indemnify

To make good a loss.

Independent Practice Association (IPA)

A health maintenance organization delivery model in which the HMO contracts with a physician organization, which, in turn, contracts with individual physicians. The IPA physicians practice in their own offices and continue to see fee-for-service patients. The HMO reimburses the IPA on a capitated basis. However, the IPA usually reimburses physicians on a fee-for-service basis. This type of system combines prepayment with the traditional means of delivering health care.

Managed Care
A general term for organizing doctors, hospitals, and other providers into groups in order to enhance the quality and the cost-effectiveness of health care. Managed care organizations (MCOs) include HMOs, PPOs, POSs, EPOs, and others.

Market Share
That part of market potential that a managed care company has captured. Usually, market share is expressed as a percentage of market potential.

Medical Group Practice
The American Group Practice Association, the American Medical Association, and the Medical Group Management Associations define medical group practice as provision of health care services by a group of at least three licensed physicians engaged in a formally organized and legally recognized entity sharing equipment, facilities, records, and personnel involved in both patient care and business management.

Medically Necessary
Covered services required to preserve and maintain the health status of a member or an eligible person in accordance with area standards of medical practice.

Multispecialty Group
A group of doctors who represent various medical specialties and who work together in a group practice.

National Committee for Quality Assurance (NCQA)
A not-for-profit organization created to improve patient care quality and health plan performance in partnership with managed care plans, purchasers, consumers, and the public sector.

Network-Model HMO
An HMO that contracts with two or more independent group practices to provide health services. It may include a few solo practices, but it is primarily organized around groups.

Open Enrollment
A period in which eligible subscribers may elect to enroll, or transfer between, available programs providing health care coverage.

Outcomes Management

A clinical outcome is the result of medical or surgical intervention or nonintervention. It is thought that, through a database of outcomes experience, caregivers will know better which treatment modalities result in consistently better outcomes for patients. Outcomes management may lead to the development of clinical protocols.

Outlier

One who does not fall within the norm. Term typically used in utilization review. A provider who uses either too many or too few services.

Out-of-Area Benefits

Coverage allowed to HMO members for emergency situations outside of the prescribed geographic area of the HMO.

Outpatient Services

Medical and other services provided by a hospital or another qualified facility, such as a mental health clinic, on other than an inpatient basis. Such services include outpatient physical therapy services, diagnostic x-ray, and laboratory tests.

Participating Provider

A health care provider who participates through a contractual arrangement with a health care service contractor, HMO, PPO, IPA, or other managed care organization.

Peer Review

A review by members of the profession regarding the quality of care provided a patient, including documentation of care (medical audit), diagnostic steps used, conclusions reached, therapy given, appropriateness of utilization (utilization review), and reasonableness of charges.

Performance Standards

Standards an individual provider is expected to meet, especially in regard to quality of care. The standards may define volume of care delivered per period. Thus, performance standards for OB/GYN may specify some or all of the following: office hours, office visits per week or month, on-call days, deliveries per year, gynecological operations per year, and the like.

Point-of-Service Plan (POS)

Also known as an open-ended HMO. POS plans encourage, but do not require, members to choose primary care physicians. As in traditional HMOs, primary care physicians act as gatekeepers when making referrals. Plan members may opt to visit non-network providers at their discretion. Subscribers choosing not to use primary care physicians must pay higher deductibles and copayments than those using network physicians.

Practice Parameters
The American Medical Association defines practice parameters as strategies for patient management developed to assist physicians in clinical decision making. They may also be referred to as practice options, practice guidelines, practice policies, or practice standards.

Preadmission Review
The practice of reviewing requests for inpatient admission prior to the patient's entering the hospital in order to ensure that the admission is medically necessary.

Preferred Provider Organization (PPO)
A health care arrangement between purchasers of care and providers that provides benefits at a reasonable cost by providing members with incentives (lower deductibles and copayments) to use providers within the network. Members who prefer to use nonpreferred physicians may do so, but only at a higher cost. Preferred providers must agree to specified fee schedules in exchange for a preferred status and are required to comply with certain utilization review guidelines.

Preauthorization
A method of monitoring and controlling utilization by evaluating the need for medical service prior to its being performed.

Quality Assurance
Activities and programs intended to ensure high-quality care in a defined medical setting. Such programs include peer or utilization review components to identify and remedy deficiencies in quality. The program must have a mechanism for assessing its effectiveness and may measure care against pre-established standards (benchmarking).

Risk
The chance or possibility of loss.

Risk Pool
A pool of money to be used for defined expenses. If money is left over at the end of the year, it is usually returned to those managing the risk.

Staff-Model HMO
An HMO that delivers health services through a physician group that is controlled by the HMO unit; most physicians are salaried employees who deal exclusively with HMO members.

Self-Insurance

An employer's or an organization's practice of assuming responsibility for health care losses of its employees. This usually entails setting up a fund against which claim payments are drawn, and claims processing is often handled through an administrative service contract with an independent organization.

Stop Loss

The point at which a third party has reinsurance to protect against an overly large single claim or an excessively high aggregate claim during a given period. Large employers who are self-insured may also purchase "reinsurance" for stop-loss purposes.

Tertiary Care

Subspecialty care usually requiring the facilities of a university-affiliated or teaching hospital that has extensive diagnostic and treatment capabilities.

Third Party

The entity that contracts with employers who want to self-insure the health of their employees. It develops and coordinates self-insurance programs, processes and pays claims, and may help locate stop-loss insurance for the employer. It can also analyze the effectiveness of the program and trace the patterns of those using the benefits.

Usual, Customary, and Reasonable (UCR)

Health insurance plans that pay a physician's full charge if it is reasonable and does not exceed the usual charges and the amount customarily charged for the service by other physicians in the same area.

Utilization Review

Also known as utilization management or utilization control, utilization review is a systematic means for reviewing and controlling patients' use of medical care services, as well as the appropriateness and quality of care. Usually involves data collection, review, and/or authorization, especially for services such as specialist referrals, emergency department use, and hospitalization.

Utilization

The patterns of use of a service or type of service within a specified period. Utilization is usually expressed in rate per unit of population at risk for a given period.

Withhold

That portion of the monthly capitation payment to physicians withheld by an HMO to create an incentive for efficient care. A physician who exceeds utilization norms does not receive the withheld amount. This system serves as a financial incentive for lower utilization. The withhold can cover all services or be specific to hospital care, laboratory usage, or specialty referrals.

Source

The Texas Medical Association Glossary of Managed Care Terminology.
http://www.texmed.org/resource_center/tma_bookstore/rc_bookmcgloss.htm